THE

Homœopathic Therapeutics

OF

DIARRHŒA,

THE
Homœopathic Therapeutics

OF

DIARRHŒA,

DYSENTERY, CHOLERA, CHOLERA MORBUS, CHOLERA INFANTUM,

AND

All Other Loose Evacuations of the Bowels.

BY

JAMES B. BELL, M.D.

THIRTEENTH EDITION.

"Science is a complement of knowledges, having, in point of form, the character of logical perfection, and, in point of matter, the character of real truth."—*Sir Wm. Hamilton.*

B. Jain Publishers (P) Ltd.
USA — EUROPE — INDIA

THE HOMEOPATHIC THERAPEUTICS OF DIARRHOEA

8th Impression: 2020

> **Note From the Publishers**
> Any information given in this book is not intended to be taken as a replacement for medical advice. Any person with a condition requiring medical attention should consult a qualified practitioner or therapist.

All rights reserved. No part of this book may be reproduced, stored in a retrieval system or transmitted, in any form or by any means, mechanical, photocopying, recording or otherwise, without any prior written permission of the publisher.

© with the publisher

Published by Kuldeep Jain for
B. JAIN PUBLISHERS (P) LTD.
D-157, Sector-63, NOIDA-201307, U.P. (INDIA)
Tel.: +91-120-4933333 • *Email:* info@bjain.com
Website: **www.bjain.com**
Registered office: 1921/10, Chuna Mandi, Paharganj,
New Delhi-110 055 (India)

Printed in India by
J.J. Offset Printers

ISBN: 978-81-319-0155-7

ACKNOWLEDGEMENT
The publisher wishes to pay a tribute of appreciation to :

DR S.P. PADIAR,
ERNAKULAM.

for providing us with the original book for printing.

PREFACE TO THE FIRST EDITION

This little work was prepared for my own use as a labor-saver, and as a receptacle for clinical observations, and for gleanings from others and from the periodicals.

It has been the work of odd moments and little remnants of time, redeemed from busy days.

Even the young physician, of a single summer's experience, must have felt the want of such a work, particularly when dealing with the frequently occurring and obstinate diarrhœas of infants. It was the difficulty of treating these that first awakened the desire to possess in one little work all that was known of our Materia Medica as applied to loose evacuations of the bowels.

It has not been intended to include every remedy that has been known to purge, but only every remedy of which enough is known, either of its stools, or conditions, or concomitants, to distinguish it from any other remedy.

But some may inquire, Why should diseases of the bowels be honored above others by a special monograph?

Those who have Bœnninghausen on Cough, on Fever, and on Headache, will not ask this question, but will desire that the work go on until we possess such special aids in the treatment of all affections that most tax the busy practitioner.

The present work is now printed because colleagues, who had seen it, desired to possess a copy—one going so far as to copy it himself,—because Mr. Tafel, who had seen it, desired to print it, and because the work had already repaid me for the time and labor it cost in the same coin, and I was therefore happy to believe that it would be of like use to others. The clinical test will be found to disclose many valuable symptoms not to be met with elsewhere, and, alas, doubtless, many errors.

The carefully collated experience of ten active years, which it contains, would indeed be better if they were twenty or thirty, but perhaps the Lord in his goodness will permit this to be added also.

It would be a grateful task to indicate throughout the work the sources from which many valuable symptoms were drawn, but this would detract from its practical character as a work of reference.

JAMES B. BELL.

AUGUSTA, Feb. 21, 1869.

AUTHOR'S PREFACE TO THE SECOND EDITION.

THE material for a new edition of this little work has been collected ever since the first was published, and such an edition has long been called for, but I do not think it would have ever seen the light had I not persuaded my friend and successor, Dr. W. T. Laird, late of Watertown, N. Y., to undertake its preparation for the press. He has also added much from his own collection of material, and to him is due the entire remodelling of the Repertory, which, in the first edition, was quite defective.

My former partner, Dr. T. M. Dillingham, had kindly made a partial revision of the work, but went abroad before its completion.

It may be necessary to add, by way of personal explanation, that my "specialty" lies in quite another direction than "Diarrhœa" or Materia Medica, and it is only as a lover of sound therapeutics that I have taken up these subjects.

Dr. Ad. Lippe has contributed two annotated copies and many suggestions, and I wish to tender my thanks to him and to all who have added any observations to its pages, as well, also, to the great numbers in the profession who have so kindly and heartily commended the book. To me its only merit is its practical application of the principles of Hahnemann, and I am rejoiced, therefore, that so many still hold firmly to those principles and seek to be guided by them.

EDITOR'S PREFACE.

In the revision of a monograph like the present work, after the lapse of twelve years, many new remedies demand recognition. These may be conveniently divided into four clases.

In the first, we place those which have been thoroughly proved and repeatedly verified in practice.

The second consists of drugs, which have also been well proved, but whose symptoms, as yet, lack clinical confirmation.

The third embraces the medicines of which we possess only fragmentary and imperfect pathogeneses. These may be styled "the suggestive remedies," and include such drugs as *Coto Bark*, *Gent. lut.*, *Geran.*, *Gnaph.*, *Hura*, *Œnothera*, *Paullinia*, etc.

The fourth division contains those remedies whose indications are derived solely *ab us in morbis*.

Of the first and second classes every remedy is plainly entitled to admission, "of which enough is known, either of its stools, or conditions, or concomitants, to distinguish it from any other remedy."

Many of the drugs in the third class are doubtless valuable, and will prove of great service when further provings, experience and observation have developed their characteristic indications. Some of them have already been successfully used in practice. Unfortunately, however, at the present time the symptoms of the majority of these remedies are too few and too uncertain to render their selection easy or to entitle them to a place in a work which is intended to be purely practical.

Remedies of the fourth class—those having no basis except empiricism—must be viewed with distrust and received with great caution.

In the second edition the same general plan has been followed as in the first, with the exception that the important symptoms are italicized, while those which are especially characteristic are printed in black type.

The term "cholera infantum" has been retained in many cases, which, according to strict pathology, would be more properly designated as entero-colitis and gastro-enteric catarrh. Although this use of the term is not defensible from a scientific standpoint, it is sanctioned to such an extent by common usage that it has been thought inexpedient to make any change.

The present edition contains over 100 pages more than the first. Thirty-two new remedies have been added, and the old ones thoroughly revised, and, in some instances, entirely rewritten.

Numerous clinical symptoms have been incorporated with the text, but only those whose genuineness is attested by trustworthy observers or which the writer has frequently verified in his own practice. Many others have been rejected on the ground of insufficient evidence.

The writer lays no claim to originality in the additions he has made to this work. His task has been mainly one of compilation. He has gleaned from our literature all that he deemed valuable, and has conscientiously endeavored to make the book as accurate and complete as possible; yet none can be more painfully aware of the many imperfections and errors of omission which it must necessarily contain. It is especially to be regretted, in this connection, that the request for contributions, printed in our journals, has met with such meagre responses from the profession; for it is only by unity of effort that we can hope to attain the best results.

The writer would gratefully acknowledge his indebtedness to Drs. W. P. Wesselhoeft and Ad. Lippe for valuable notes and suggestions; to Prof. E. A. Farrington for important information, and also for his kind permission to make free use of very complete notes of his lectures on Materia Medica; and to Dr. F. F. Laird for assistance in preparing the manuscript.

AUGUSTA, ME., March, 1881.

W. T. LAIRD, M. D.

PREFACE TO THIRD EDITION.

THIS book has been most thoroughly revised, with the earnest purpose of making it as nearly complete as possible. Four remedies of little importance have been omitted, viz.: *Cactus*, *Euphorb.*, *Opuntia* and *Castoreum*, and five of much value have been added, viz.: *Acetic acid*, *Crotalus*, *Angustura*, *Carbolic acid* and *Valeriana*.

The more closely one follows the principles discovered by Hahnemann the more priceless appears the legacy which he has left us. We have no occasion to join in the pursuit of new, but speedily discarded drugs, lauded first as specifics, then thrown over for their failures and harmful effects. We are able at once, by proving and observation, to rightly estimate and use the new as well as the old remedies, and the knowledge thus acquired will be just as valuable centuries hence as now, and so we work on with the solemn joy of those whose work will never cease to bless mankind while there remain any sick to be healed.

Dr. Samuel A. Kimball, author of the Monograph on Gonorrhœa, has given faithful and most valuable assistance in this revision, and Drs. J.

G. Allen and W. Jefferson Guernsey have furnished annotated copies of the earlier edition. Many others also have contributed observations and suggestions, to all of whom most cordial thanks are tendered.

JAMES B. BELL.

BOSTON, June, 1888.

PREFACE TO FOURTH EDITION.

THE most that can be said as a preface to a fourth edition, is that a thorough revision, and re-revision, and a renewed comparison with all the Materia Medica now available, reveals but few changes to make, and no remedies to add or to omit.

ALLEN'S SYMPTOM REGISTER gives four hundred and twenty-five remedies as having diarrhœa, and KNERR'S REPERTORY of the GUIDING SYMPTOMS a much smaller list, but none of them, not already included in this book, are suited for a place in it, either because the proving is indefinite, or because the diarrhœa is simply accessory to a larger and more important group of symptoms (as in *Diadema* in Intermittent fever, or *Asteria rubens* in Epilepsy, or *Arum triphyllum* in Typhoid or Scarlet fever) and is not particularly well defined in itself. It would seem, therefore, that this little work is now as complete as it can well be made, for at least some time to come.

Homœopathy is not making that kind of "progress" that renders a whole medical library obsolete every ten years, but instead of that, is all the time laying up in its storehouse treasures new and old.

JAMES B. BELL.

178 COMMONWEALTH AVE., Boston, Oct., 1896.

INTRODUCTION.

CHARACTER AND OBJECT OF THE WORK.

This work is intended to apply to all loose evacuations of the bowels, and to describe them, their aggravations and ameliorations, with their immediate accompaniments and general accompanying symptoms.

The character of the stool is used as an adjective, and after it the "stool" is always to be understood. The semicolon stands for it.

Under the head of aggravations and ameliorations those influences are given which affect the stool, and also those which act as excited causes of the attack. When referring to other symptoms, they will be found indicated in parentheses.

The concomitants of the stool have been studied and observed with much care.

The general accompaniments include all the symptoms that occur during the attack.

Under each of the best known remedies some symptoms will be found italicized. These, it will be understood, are the symptoms which have been most frequently observed, and which also serve to most sharply distinguish that remedy from others. The more of these emphasized symptoms we have under any one remedy the easier the selection. The sooner we are able by careful observation to emphasize symptoms under all our remedies, the more we shall perfect our art. It should be the self-appointed task of every Homœopathic physician to confirm, and define, and add to the symptoms of all our remedies, but more especially of those that are but little known. Many of that class will be found in this book, some of which have many symptoms of clear and distinctive character, derived from provings, but whose relative and positive value awaits clinical determination. If those who use this book will add the fruits of their observations by underlining and writing-in symptoms, they will be gladly incorporated in a future edition, should any be required.

The remarks, which follow nearly every remedy, should be understood as embodying only the personal opinions of the writer, whether confirming or contradicting what may have been published by others. It is hoped that they may sometimes aid in the selection of the remedy, but they are of wholly subordinate authority to the text.

THE SELECTION OF THE REMEDY.

All who subscribe to the law of similars agree that the problem in each case is to find a remedy whose symptoms are most closely similar to the case in hand. This problem finds a somewhat different solution, however, in different classes of mind.

One class thinks the solution is found in a similitude to the pathological state. If able to diagnose hyperæmia, hyperæsthesia, ulceration, plastic exudation, atony, atrophy, hypertrophy, and so on through the catalogue, this seems to them sufficient. They have only then to diagnose a remedy producing a similar state. This has a great fascination for some excellent minds, because it seems to utilize the splendid developments of Allopathy in this direction, and connect them directly with therapeutics.

Another, and growing class, believes that those who stop here will never comprehend the true genius of Homœopathy. The demand for exactness, minuteness and delicacy of observation in all branches of science was never greater. The same is true of Homœopathic Therapeutics. Those who are ardently following in this direction soon discover that the selection of the remedy requires, so to speak, two similars, viz.: one corresponding to the general symptoms, or those which bring it into relation to the pathological state to be treated, and one corresponding to the special and characteristic symptoms, or those which bring it into relation with the individual case to be treated.

To illustrate: a patient has stools consisting of bloody mucus, small and frequent, with tenesmus. We diagnose dysentery; hyperæmia and inflammation of the mucous membrane of the colon, with exudation of blood and secretion of mucus. Forty-four volunteers stand ready, armed and equipped with a similar pathological condition. But we want but one, and how shall we learn which one? We must be more exact, and discover that our patient has restlessness, dry heat and much thirst. Our volunteers are now reduced to three; but still too many. Applying our magnifying-glass again, we observe a recent exposure to cold, dry wind, and a flushed face becoming pale, with faintness on rising, and now we have the man we want.

It becomes evident, therefore, that the individualizing symptoms possess the greater value, and are, indeed, indispensable to a certain selection.

It should be noticed, further, that these distinguishing symptoms are of all kinds and qualities, from the most purely objective and pathological, to the most subjective and delicate complaints which the organism is capable of uttering. As instances of the former may be cited, the green frothy stools of *Magn. c.*, the dark acid urine of *Benz. ac.*, the blue varices of *Mur. ac.*, and of the latter, the aggravation from hearing water run, of *Hydroph.*, from sudden depressing emotions, of *Gels.*, and the relief, from cold food and drink, of *Phos.*

But whatever the character of these symptoms, in this particular, it is to be observed that they are hardly ever obstrusive enough to thrust themselves upon the notice of an unobserving man, and that they often require a patience and acuteness of observation hardly excelled by astronomers, microscopists and other followers of natural science.

This mode of diagnosing the remedy is also in exact accordance with that pursued in other sciences. The chemist would be thought hardly worthy of his title who should attempt to recognize *Arsenic* by its cruder properties of color, weight, or taste. He must be familiar with its most delicate and characteristic tests and reactions. He does not ignore the other properties, yet it is only after applying the characteristic tests that he will give an authoritative decision, and on these he will rely, even in cases involving weighty questions of human guilt or innocence.

But now the question arises, and it is a very important and practical one: suppose we find that the only remedy for a given case, that corresponds to the peculiar and individualizing symptoms, is one that has never been known to cause the pathological state under which our patient suffers. The answer is, that we may safely infer that the remedy does possess also the general and organic symptoms of the case, and that it will remove them, together with the distinguishing indications.

Thus has our Materia Medica been enriched by at least one-fourth of the most positive and valuable pathological symptoms which we possess. Thus, for example, have we learned that *Bry.*, *Ars.*, *Rhus*, *Bap.*, etc., have ulceration of Peyer's glands in their pathogenesis; that *Hep.*, *Lach.* and *Lyc.* produce pseudo-membraneous exudation; that *Spong.* causes and cures plastic endocarditis; or that (and a fact now published for the first time and obtained purely by observing the characteristic symptoms) *Puls.* and *Sep.* are known to cause and cure trachoma or granular conjunctivitis.

Yet some affect to sneer at this method, and only a little time ago the author had the honor to acquire an enviable title,* because he had observed the power of *Podoph.* to cure true pneumonia when selected by some characteristic symptoms, although it has never been known to produce that condition.

Yet here, too, we are following closely the example of the chemist, who from the yellow band in the spectrum is able to assert that there is sodium in the sun, or from the lines in the spectrum of the Dürkheim spring-water is able to declare that a new metal is there. He does not hesitate to attribute form, weight, malleability and other metallic properties to the stranger, long before he is able to possess himself of a little bar of Indium.

Our conclusion, then, is, that the problem of selection is solved by seeking the remedy which

---

*"Podophyllum Bell."

possesses the physical and diagnostic symptoms of the case, and which corresponds also to the special, distinguishing and peculiar symptoms which mark the individual case. And further, if a remedy is found that possesses distinctly the latter symptoms, but not, so far as is known, the former, we may conclude safely that it does possess the former, and administer it with confidence.

THE ADMINISTRATION OF THE REMEDY

In the present state of our science upon this point, each can only contribute the fruits of his own observation.

The writer began the practice of medicine with the preconceived idea strongly fixed in his mind, that, while the thirtieth potency might be useful and perhaps the best for chronic and nervous affections, the lower and even crude preparations would prove more satisfactory for acute affections and particularly for diseases of the bowels.

Hard experience has taught him the contrary, and "though convinced against his will," he is not "of the same opinion still."

There is indeed a somewhat prevalent opinion, that the strength of the dose makes up for want of due care or knowledge in selection.

This may be stated in mathematical terms as follows: If the thirtieth potency of *Ars.* is equal to a complete knowledge of the drug, one-fifth of a grain of *Arsenious acid* is equal to complete ignorance of it. Stated in this, its true form, we grant it.

Personally, our experience has been most satisfactory with the use of the twelfth, fifteenth, thirtieth, two hundredth, and often higher potencies, of our remedies, administered in water, and repeated every one to six hours according to the urgency of the symptoms, and suspended as soon as decided improvement appeared. If the same remedy was needed to be resumed again, it has seemed to do better in a higher potency, but on this point we cannot yet speak with entire assurance.

We have not been able to perceive that age or sex or habits (we might add color, race or order in natural history) form any element in the choice of the dose. All classes have been found to respond favorably to the high potencies. As regards temperament, we cannot speak with equal positiveness, but we have no certain testimony proving it to form an exception.

Homœopathic Therapeutics.

PART I.

The Remedies and their Indications.

1. ACETIC ACID.

Stools: Liquid; Frequent; Undigested; Very offensive; Painful (liquid stools); Exhausting.

Aggravation: In the morning: In phthisical subjects: In typhoid: In ascites.

Accompaniments: Intense thirst, and water does not seem to disagree, even when taken in large quantities. Wants *nothing* but fluids. Complains much of the stomach. The abdomen is sometimes swollen very much. Feet and legs often swell. Has restless, sleepless, uncomfortable nights. Great emaciation. Great debility. Pale, waxen skin. Violent thirst in diarrhœa, with swelling of legs and feet, in phthisis. Thirstlessness in diarrhœa in latter stages of typhus and typhoid fever. No thirst in croup.

The most characteristic of **Acetic acid** is the thirst.

We are indebted to Dr. H. N. Guernsey for most of the symptoms.

2. ACONITE.

Stools: *Watery;* Black; *Green like chopped spinach;* Bilious; Corrosive; *Bloody, slimy, mucous; Small;* Brown, small, painful; **Frequent** (dysenteric stool); Involuntary (when passing flatus).

Aggravation: In summer, with hot days and cold nights: *After getting wet:* After being overheated: After exposure to cold, dry wind, or a draught: After anger or fright: After suppressed perspiration: At night: After eating fruit: In infants.

Amelioration: After eating warm soup—(pains).

Before Stool: Cutting pains: Nausea and sweat: Anguish.

During Stool: Cutting pains: **Tenesmus:** Sweat: Much flatus (with watery stools).

After Stool: Relief, except from anguish, nausea and sweat, which may continue.

Accompaniments: *Anxiety; Fear of death.* **Restlessness.** *Vertigo or fainting on rising up*, with paleness; face flushed when lying. Bitter taste of everything except water. Lips dry, dark. **Unquenchable thirst.** Nausea. Vomiting: of blood; of blood and mucus; of bile; of what has been drunk with profuse sweat. Sensation of a cold stone in the stomach. Distended abdomen sensitive to the touch. Abdomen very hot. Violent pains (cutting) in the abdomen. Colic, of infants, which no position relieves (with bilious stool). Rheumatic pains in head, nape of neck and shoulders. Urine high-colored, scanty and pungent, without sediment.

Sleeplessness. **General dry heat. Full, hard, very quick pulse.** Internal shuddering, with dry, hot skin, and tendency to uncover. Sweat on the covered parts.

In Cholera: Hippocratic countenance; face bluish; lips black; expression of terror and imbecility; cold limbs with blue nails. Collapse.

Acon. is especially useful in the very beginning of acute diseases of the bowels, and is then often able to cut short dysentery and even cholera morbus without any other remedy. It is also a valuable intercurrent in dysentery, when **Merc. cor.**, although indicated, fails to relieve. It closely resembles **Dulc.** and is followed well by that drug, also by **Bell.**

Abuse of **Acon.** calls for **Sulph.**

3. ÆSCULUS HIPPOCASTANUM.

Stools: *Papescent;* Mushy; Slimy; White; light brown; First part black and hard, last part white as milk; Bloody and slimy (with hæmorrhoids); Watery, painless in P. M.; Thin, yellow.

Before Stool: Rumbling in bowels with cutting about navel: Sudden urging: Passing of flatus.

During Stool: *Severe lumbar and sacral pains:* Weakness: Tenesmus: Unpleasant sensation in rectum and anus: Fetid flatus.

After Stool: Relief of pain in abdomen: Pain in abdomen and eructations tasting of the ingesta.

Accompaniments: Gloomy and despondent. Irritable. Dull frontal headache. Dryness of posterior nares, fauces and throat. Colicky pains and rumbling in abdomen. *Excessive dryness, heat and itching in rectum; rectum feels as if filled with small sticks;* mucous membrane feels swollen, obstructing the passing of fæces. Soreness, burning, fulness and itching of anus, with prolapsed feeling. *Painful, burning, purple hæmorrhoids.* **Violent backache in sacro-lumbar region, aggravated by walking or stooping. Pain across sacro-iliac symphysis with feeling as if back would break.**

Æsculus will prove serviceable in the chronic diarrhœa of patients, who suffer from hæmorrhoidal troubles, associated with the severe lumbar and sacral pains characteristic of this remedy.

4. ÆTHUSA CYNAPIUM.

Stools: Bilious, *light yellow* and *greenish* (liquid); Greenish-gray; *Green mucous; Bloody mucous;* Undigested; Profuse; Inodorous (greenish stools); Watery, slimy.

Aggravation: In the morning (after rising):

THEIR INDICATIONS.

In children: In summer: During dentition: Shortly after a meal or at night (undigested).

Before Stool: Pinching and cutting pains in the abdomen.

During Stool: Tenesmus, often violent: Painful contractions.

After Stool: Unsatisfied urging to stool: violent tenesmus: *Exhaustion: Drowsiness.*

Accompaniments: Irritability, bad humor, especially afternoons and in the open air. Sensation as though the head, and other parts, were in a vise. Face pale or flushed, altered; collapsed, with an expression of anguish. Aphthæ. Constant thirst. *Intolerance of milk. Sudden and violent vomiting immediately after nursing; milk is thrown up just as it was swallowed,* **or in curds so large as to almost choke the child;** sometimes it looks *oily and greenish.* Vomiting without nausea; of *greenish mucus;* of frothy, milk-white substance. *Vomiting is followed by exhaustion and deep sleep, but child nurses again as soon as it wakes.* Spasmodic hiccough. Crying. Drawing up the feet. Painful contractions in stomach.

Stupor. Spasms: thumbs clenched; eyes turned down; pupils fixed, dilated; eyes staring; foam at the mouth; red face; locked jaw; pulse small, hard and quick. Surface of body cold and covered with clammy sweat. Drowsiness with chilliness. Violent startings during sleep. Great prostration.

Æthus. is suitable to a severe form of cholera infantum. It will usually be hardly able to complete the cure alone, but will need to be followed by an antipsoric; most frequently by **Psor., Sep.,** or **Sulph.**

5. AGARICUS.

Stool: *Thin, yellow, fecal and slimy;* Watery; *Grass-green;* Bilious; Bloody; *Fetid;* Smelling like carrion.

Aggravation: In the morning after rising and eating: In wet weather (general condition): After eating.

Before Stool: Pinching and cutting in the abdomen: *Sudden violent urging:* Painful straining in the rectum.

During Stool: The pains continue, with nausea: Rumbling and fermentation in the abdomen: Crampy colic with *emission of much flatus:* Painful drawing-in of the stomach and abdomen: Smarting in the anus: Burning soreness and cutting in anus: Sweat: Pains in loins to legs.

After Stool: Smarting in the anus: Cutting in the rectum: Biting and burning in anus: Straining in rectum: Griping in hypogastrium: Distension of abdomen: Heaviness in abdomen and around navel: Pains in chest: Pains in loins to legs: Headache worse.

Accompaniments: Mental excitability. Dulness almost amounting to idiocy. Merry, loquacious, delirium. Children morose, self-willed, stubborn. Slow in learning to walk and talk. Vertigo in the morning; in the open air; in the bright sun. White-coated tongue. Acrid, offensive smell from the mouth, like horse-radish. Passage of much flatus, smelling like garlic. Sleepiness in the daytime, after eating. Burning, itching, red spots on the skin, which fade away as the diarrhœa improves.

There has been but little clinical experience with **Agar.** in diarrhœa. It resembles **Natr. sulph.** in its symptoms, also **Baryta carb.**, and is especially useful in chronic diarrhœa.

6. ALOE.

Stools: *Yellow fecal; Bloody, jelly-like mucous;* Green mucous; *Transparent jelly-like mucous;* Yellowish, greenish, or bright yellow, bilious; Gray; Profuse with jelly-like lumps; Profuse watery, containing lumps looking like frog spawn; Brownish, slimy; Bloody water; Gushing; Hot; Undigested;—*Involuntary (when expelling flatus, or urine, when walking, standing, or after eating);* Small (dysenteric stool); Papescent; Lumpy; *Semi-liquid; Watery;* Moderately offensive (yellow, watery stools); Foul smelling (bloody mucous stools).

Aggravation: *In hot, damp weather:* In the afternoon, evening and night: *Early in the morning, driving one out of bed: From 5 to 10 A. M.: After acids* (vinegar): After chagrin: After overheating: After cold taken in a damp room: From motion: *When walking or standing: After eating: After drinking: When passing urine.*

Amelioration: From ale (pains in the anus): By bending double and by passing flatus (colic).

Before Stool: *Difficulty of retaining the stool:* Urging to stool, only hot flatus passes giving relief: Urging, violent, quickly passing, frequent, *with feeling of fulness and weight in the pelvis, as if the rectum were full of fluid, which feels heavy as though it would fall out:* **Feeling of weakness and loss of power of sphincter ani: Sense of insecurity in the rectum,** *as if the stool would escape* **when passing flatus,** or urine: Burning and cutting in rectum: *Sensation of a plug wedged between symphysis pubis and coccyx:* Colic: Burning heat and prickling in the intestines: *Pain around the navel*: Much flatus: Rumbling of flatus: Twisting and griping pain in upper abdomen and around navel, relieved by bending double: Great cutting, griping, excruciating pains in right and lower portion of abdomen: Rush of blood to the head.

During Stool: Urging: Cutting and tearing in the abdomen extorting cries: Cutting and griping continues: *Hunger: Heat in the rectum and anus: Violent tenesmus: Much flatus:* Heat of the whole body: Congestion to head and face: Distress in region of liver: Chilliness: Fainting.

After Stool: Feeling as if still more would come: *Swelling, burning, weight,* and itching in the anus: *Large and prominent hæmorrhoids, tender, hot, relieved by cold water: Abdominal pains usually relieved:* Cutting about the navel and griping, sometimes continues: *Prostration: Fainting: Profuse, clammy sweat.*

Accompaniments: Dissatisfied and angry about himself when in pain. Constant headache with slight nausea. Lips red, and tongue dry and red, with much thirst. Generally, *good appetite*. Desire for juicy things; apples; beer. Aversion to meat. Bitter taste. Pain in hypochondria, with painful weakness in legs. Heat, fulness, pressure and tenderness in the abdomen and *region of the liver*. Griping pains in the abdomen, relieved by bending double, with urging to stool, nothing but flatus being passed. Shooting and boring pains around navel increased by pressure. Intense griping pain across the lower part of the abdomen, especially on the right side. Lower part of abdomen swollen and sensitive to pressure. Cutting and pinching pains in rectum and loins. Much flatus moving about in the abdomen, more in the left side. Pain in bowels after eating. *Loud gurgling in the abdomen as water running out of a bottle.* Distended abdomen. Flatus smells very badly, and causes burning in the rectum. Urine generally profuse. Involuntary urination. Heaviness and numbness of the thighs. Chilliness when leaving the fire. Repugnance to open air, which, nevertheless, relieves.

Aloe is one of our most valuable remedies for both diarrhœa and dysentery. It is undoubtedly a deeply acting antipsoric and of great value in chronic diarrhœa. The symptoms are marked and unmistakable, as given above. Contrary to what might be expected, the peculiar gurgling in the abdomen is often found with the dysenteric stool, when **Aloe** is indicated. The good appetite is most frequently met with in children. The hæmorrhoids differ from those of **Brom.** in the relief from cold water, and from those of **Muriatic acid,** which are relieved by warm water and greatly aggravated by cold water locally applied. It has many symptoms like **Sulphur** and is nearly as important a remedy.

7. ALUMINA.

Stools: Thin fecal; Black, *bloody;* Green, *watery;* Corrosive; *Expulsion difficult.*

Aggravation: After constipation: After dinner: After lead-poisoning: During typhoid fever: In dry weather: When walking: When urinating: *On alternate days* (general condition): From pap and artificial food (children).

Amelioration: After short sleep: From warm applications (colic): In open air (general condition).

Before Stool: Colic.

During Stool: Colic: Tenesmus (with bloody, scanty stools): Burning in the rectum: Involuntary urination: Dropping of blood: Heat and tenderness of bowels.

After Stool: Usually relief: Sometimes the colic continues: Throbbing in the back: Soreness of anus: Involuntary urination.

THEIR INDICATIONS.

Accompaniments: Seriousness. Changeable mood. Apprehensive, melancholy and tearful or irritable and fretful. Inclined to be hysterical. Reeling vertigo in the morning, with faintness or nausea. *Strabismus from weakness of internal rectus* (during dentition). Feeling of constriction in œsophagus when swallowing: Capricious appetite. Aversion to meat. Desire for chalk, *starch*, clean white rags, charcoal, cloves, acids, ground coffee, tea-grounds, dirt, dry rice, and other unnatural and indigestible substances. Faintness at the stomach, relieved by satisfying the depraved cravings. *Always worse after eating potatoes*. Palpitation of heart with large and small beats intermingled. Violent colic. **Urine can only be passed with the stool,** *or must stand up to urinate and then sit down to defecate*. Sensation of weakness of sphincter ani. General debility. *Chlorosis*. **Great dryness of all the mucous membranes. Dryness and harshness of skin with absence of perspiration.**

Alum. is sometimes useful in acute diarrhœa and, possibly, dysentery, when the difficult expulsion of stool and urine exists. It is more frequently indicated in chronic diarrhœa accompanying chlorosis in slender delicate girls, with the depraved appetite and the aggravation on alternate days. With these symptoms, a brilliant cure may be expected, including the chlorosis, if the remedy be not given too low and too frequently

8. AMMONIUM MURIATICUM.

Stools: Green, thin, mucous (slimy); Yellow fecal and slimy; White and undigested; Green and watery; Yellow and bloody, watery, or slimy; Like scrapings of meat; Copious (watery); Copious of coagulated blood; Constipation alternating with diarrhœa.

Aggravation: In the morning (green slimy stools): *During the menses:* After meals: During the day: Walking in open air (nausea).

Before Stool: Violent urging: *Pain about the navel*.

During Stool: Tenesmus: Pain in the rectum: Burning in rectum: Discharge of blood: Pain in abdomen, back and limbs: Pain in small of back.

After Stool: Tenesmus: Pain in abdomen, and soreness as if bruised: Burning in rectum: Sore pustules near the anus.

Accompaniments: Fretfulness. Face bloated, red, flushes easily. Bitter taste in the mouth, and bitter eructations passing off after eating something. Loss of appetite. Nausea, after dinner and when walking in the open air. Pinching in abdomen, hindering inspiration. Much rumbling and emission of flatus. Itching soreness of the rectum, several pustules being formed at the side of it. Ebullitions of blood, violent throbbing in arteries, with anxiety and feeling of paralytic weakness. Bruised pain in the whole body in the morning after rising.

Amm. m. is especially adapted to fat, sluggish people, with adipose tissue well developed on the trunk, while the legs are disproportionately small. It is useful for chronic diarrhœa occurring during the menses, when the other symptoms correspond. Many of the symptoms resemble those of **Aloe** but are milder. The green mucous stool may render it useful in infantile diarrhœa, but experience with it in this affection is yet wanting.

9. ANGUSTURA.

Stools: Mucous; Yellow; Whitish; Slimy; Copious (thin stools).

Aggravation: In morning: During day: At night.

Before Stool: Cutting in abdomen and nausea: Sensation in rectum as if it would protrude.

During Stool: Painful tenesmus: Distension of hæmorrhoidal veins: Burning in rectum.

After Stool: Shivering passing over the face, with gooseflesh: Feeling as if more would come.

Accompaniments: Wants one thing, now another, refused when offered. Desires nothing but warm drinks. Thirst without desire for drink. Aversion to solids. Nausea in the morning. Pains in abdomen worse from warm milk, and caused by it. Fermentation and rumbling in abdomen. Offensive flatus. Urging in rectum, with crawling over the face. Pressing, contracting, tickling in rectum and anus. Stool not so thin as one would suppose from the diarrhœic feeling. Chronic diarrhœa, with debility and loss of flesh.

10. ANTIMONIUM CRUDUM.

Stools: Watery; Often profuse; Alternating with constipation; *Undigested, containing fecal lumps or hard lumps of curdled milk;* Excoriating; Mucous; Yellowish, offensive.

Aggravation: *After acids (vinegar, sour wine): After overheating: After cold bathing:* After cold water or cold food: *In aged persons:* During pregnancy: At night: Early in the morning: From pork: From summer heat: After nursing: In childbed: After deranging the stomach: After a debauch: Morning (mucous stools).

Before Stool: Cutting pains.

During Stool: Pain in the rectum: (Protrusion of the rectum).

After Stool: Prolapsus recti: Excoriation of anus.

Accompaniments: Sentimental or distrustful mood. *Children cannot bear being touched or looked at.* Fear of company. Pale face. *Nostrils and corners of mouth sore, cracked and crusty.* Ptyalism, with saltish taste. Thirst, worse at night, or thirstlessness. **Tongue coated white.** *Violent vomiting; bitter; of bile; of slimy mucus; renewed on taking food or drink.* Greenish vomiting soon after nursing. *Vomiting of sour curds. Vomiting continues after nausea ceases.* Disinclination to nurse. Frequent eructations. Eructations tasting of food. Cutting in abdomen. Desire for acids. Frequent and profuse urine, with reddish sediment. Constant secretion of a yellowish-white mucus at the anus.

The gastric symptoms of **Antimon. crud.** predominate. The vomiting differs from that of **Acon., Ars., Verat.,** and other remedies, in the absence of severe thirst and in the white-coated tongue. From want of attention to these distinctions, this remedy is often overlooked, when it would bring speedy relief.

11. ANTIMONIUM TARTARICUM.

Stools: Light, brownish-yellow, fecal; Watery; Mucous; Bloody; Green, slimy, mucous; Frequent; Profuse; Thin, bilious; Liquid, greenish; Slimy like yeast; Of cadaverous smell.

Aggravation: During exanthemata: During pneumonia: In drunkards: By pressure and bending double (colic): After taking cold in summer: At night.

Before Stool: Violent shifting of flatulence, without distension of the abdomen: *Sharp, cutting colic:* Nausea.

During Stool: Tenesmus: Nausea: Colic: Heat at the anus.

After Stool: Relief of pains: Tenesmus: Burning at the anus.

Accompaniments: Great irritability. Child cannot bear to be touched or looked at. Headache. Desire for acids, fruits. *Thirst for cold* *drinks*, with desire to drink often and but little at a time, or thirstlessness. Aversion to milk. Eructations smelling like rotten eggs. **Continuous, anxious nausea, straining to vomit, with perspiration on the forehead.** *Worse lying on left side, relieved lying on right side.* Vomiting of food; of greenish, watery, frothy substances; of mucus; *with great effort. Vomiting is accompanied by trembling of the hands and fainting; and is followed by great languor, drowsiness, loathing, desire for cooling things; pale, sunken face; dim, swimming eyes.*

Violent and painful urging to urinate, with scanty or bloody discharge.

Palpitation of the heart. *Much yawning and stretching. Drowsiness. Somnolency.* Jerking up of the limbs during sleep. Great prostration, cold sweat and thready pulse.

Although not of frequent use in diarrhœa, **Tartar emet.** will repay careful study. **Veratrum** has doubtless been given many times where the choice should have fallen on this remedy, as the colic, desires and vomiting are quite similar.

Tartar emet., however, has more drowsiness and itching of the muscles than **Verat.**

12. APIS MELLIFICA.

Stools: *Greenish, yellowish, slimy, mucous; Yellow, watery;* Yellow fecal; Clear (colorless) watery; Black watery (copious); Yellow brown; Gelatinous, mucous; Brownish, watery or bloody;

Looking like tomato sauce; Bloody watery; Olive-green, containing bright red lumps; Whitish; *Bloody mucous (mixed with fecal);* Bloody; Containing flakes of pus; *Offensive* (watery stool); *Painless* (slimy mucous, or greenish-yellow); Painless (mornings); Brassy smelling; Smelling like carrion; **Involuntary, with every motion, as though the anus stood open** (yellow fecal and slimy); **Constant oozing from anus, of which the patient is unconscious;** Frequent.

Aggravation: *In the morning:* In the forenoon: From acids: In a warm room: From motion: After eating: During dentition: During typhoid fever: Returning at the same hour.

Before Stool: Sudden darting pain in the rectum: Much rumbling of flatus: Passage of flatus: Urging.

During Stool: Urging: Griping: Tenesmus: Rawness and soreness in the anus: Bruised feeling in the intestines: Pain as if bowels were squeezed to pieces: Much flatus: Frequent painful urination: Pinching: Nausea: Vomiting: Frontal headache: Backache.

After Stool: Rawness in the anus: Heat and throbbing in rectum, with sensation as if plugged: Tenesmus with passage of blood: Faint, exhausted.

Accompaniments: Inability to fix the thoughts on any subject. *Head hot, especially the back of the head. Boring of the head back into the pillow.* Anterior fontanelle very large and *sunken*.

Eyeballs rolled upward. Eyes have a reddish tint. Face pale, waxy, œdematous. Pain in eyeball and forehead. Tongue, dry, shining, cracked, sore, with vesicles along the edges. No appetite. **Little or no thirst;** or insatiable thirst, drinking often and but little at a time. Nausea. Vomiting of food, of bile, of a thin, bitter or sour fluid. Abdomen bloated, with flatulency and rumbling. **Bruised, sore feeling of abdominal walls, with excessive tenderness,** *felt when sneezing or upon the least pressure.* Burning in the abdomen. Rawness, smarting and soreness of anus. *Urine frequent and profuse,* or scanty, or suppressed. Strangury. Labored respiration. Disturbed sleep, with muttering. Drowsiness. Dry, hot skin. **Stupor interrupted by occasional piercing shrieks.** Hands blue and cold. Cold forearms. Increasing prostration. Emaciation. Indescribable feeling of weakness. Anasarca. Ascites.

In infantile diarrhœa and cholera infantum **Apis** is one of our most precious remedies, corresponding to a low and dangerous condition. The absence of thirst, existing with a dry tongue and dry hot skin, is sufficiently striking to prevent confounding it with other remedies with similar stools. Still more characteristic is the bruised soreness of the abdominal walls. This is always present. Even when hydrocephaloid ensues, and the previously distended abdomen becomes sunken and flabby, there is still the same intolerance of the slightest pressure. When œdema is present it will be most frequently found in the feet and genitals.

13. ARGENTUM NITRICUM.

Stools: *Green mucous*, **like chopped spinach in flakes;** *Turning green after remaining on diaper;* Bright yellow; Greenish-yellow; Creamy; Dark, watery mucous; Bloody; Bloody mucous; Brown liquid; Slimy; *Masses of epithelial substance, connected by muco-lymph, red, green, shreddy, thin, unshapely strips or shaggy lumps; Frequent; Fetid* (green mucous and brown liquid); Sour; Like rotten eggs; Scanty (watery mucous); Painless (bloody mucous); Involuntary; *Undigested;* Excoriating; Alternating with constipation; **Expelled forcibly with much spluttering.**

Aggravation: *At night: After midnight:* At 6 A. M.: After rich food: **After eating freely of sugar or candy: From drinking:** After weaning: After breakfast: During dentition: Early in the morning: After eating (pains in stomach): From exalted imagination.

Amelioration: After eating, and after acid food (nausea): *From eructation:* Bending double: Pressing stomach on a chair (colic).

Before Stool: Colic: Emission of flatus: Sudden urging.

During Stool: Colic: Urging: *Emission of much noisy flatus:* Tenesmus: Severe bearing down in the hypogastrium: Nausea: *Cramping* *pain in the rectum:* Burning, constriction and sore pain in left side of abdomen.

After Stool: Relief of pain: Vomiting.

Accompaniments: Time seems to pass very slowly. Aversion to being looked at or touched. Wants to be let alone. Head feels enlarged or as if in a vise. Boring pain in left frontal eminence, relieved by hard pressure. Face pale, sunken, old-looking, brown, sallow, wrinkled. Lips and mouth dry and viscid, with little or no thirst. Gums tender and bleed easily, but seldom swollen or painful. Desire for sugar in the evening. Teeth sensitive to cold or acid substances, with constant dull grumbling. *Nausea, with loud eructations. Ineffectual efforts to eructate, causing strangulation, which is finally relieved by loud belching; the paroxysm is preceded by yawning and followed by exhaustion and deep sleep.* Violent vomiting of glassy tenacious mucus, capable of being drawn into threads. Vomiting of greenish water and milk. Burning, constriction and soreness in left side of the abdomen. Sudden stitches through the abdomen on moving. Cannot bear pressure of clothes about the hypochondria. Much flatulent colic. Urine profuse and watery, or *scanty and almost suppressed*. Spasms of respiratory muscles, with constriction of the chest and such intense dyspnœa that even a handkerchief before the face impedes respiration; can neither drink nor talk; intolerable agony. Weight in the back when standing. Uneasy sleep. *Drowsiness or stupor*, with *dilated pupils*.

Nervous restlessness with trembling and long, deep, sighing breathing. *Tremulous weakness* and debility, with much vertigo. Debility felt mostly in legs. Chilliness. Feeling of expansion in various parts. *Great emaciation*. Child looks old and dried up like a mummy.

Sudden and severe attacks of cholera infantum, with the characteristic stools, in children who are very fond of sugar, and who have eaten too much of it, will find their remedy in **Argent. nit.**

This drug is also likely to prove useful in advanced cases of dysentery with ulceration.

14. ARNICA MONTANA.

Stools· Slimy *mucous; Brown fermented (like yeast);* Undigested; *Bloody; Purulent;* Papescent; Dark, bloody mucous; *Frothy;* Thin fecal; Large, fetid (fecal); Yellow; Painless; Sourish smelling; **Offensive;** Frequent; Small; *Involuntary (during sleep);* Long intervals between (dysenteric).

Aggravation: *After mechanical injuries:* From motion: From lying on the left side: In typhoid fever: During gastric fever.

Amelioration: By passing flatus (pain in abdomen).

Before Stool: Feeling of fermentation in bowels: Frequent urging: Distension of abdomen: Severe pressure at anus.

During Stool: Urging: Tenesmus: Sore,

bruised pain in the abdomen: Cutting in intestines: Rumbling and pressure in abdomen: Distressing tenesmus in rectum and anus, and even of the bladder: Bruised pain in back.

After Stool: Relief of tenesmus and urging: Relief of pain in abdomen: Obliged to lie down.

Accompaniments: Head hotter than body, or head and breast warm, abdomen and limbs cold. Pale, sunken face. *Sour, bitter, slimy or putrid taste. Aversion to food, especially meat and broth.* Desire for vinegar; for spirits. *Thirsty, but does not know what he wants, for all drinks are alike offensive.* Constant sense of repletion in stomach, with nausea. Vomiting of what has been drunk. Hard swelling in right side of abdomen, with sharp, stitching pains when touched, relieved by passing flatus. Loud rumbling in the bowels. *Tympanitic distension of abdomen. Frequent eructations: bitter, sour, or smelling like rotten eggs. Putrid flatus.* Tenesmus of bladder, with frequent, unsuccessful urging to urinate. *Urine scanty, and stains linen yellowish-brown; sometimes passed involuntarily. Fetid breath. Offensive sweat. Great drowsiness and weakness. Stupor.* Petechiæ and ecchymoses. **The whole body feels sore and bruised, and is sensitive to touch.** *Bed feels too hard. Restless, constantly changing position.* Weakness obliging one to lie down.

Arnica has not a wide application in bowel affections, but the symptoms are clear and the selection easy. The marked gastric derangement is peculiar and characteristic.

15. ARSENICUM.

Stools: *Thick, dark green mucous;* White, slimy, bloody mucous; Fluid fecal and bloody, chocolate-colored; Slimy mucous; *Brown mucous;* Black mucous; Yellow, like stirred eggs; *Bloody; Dark or black, watery or fluid;* Yellow, watery; Purulent; Undigested; Alternating with constipation; *Frequent; Scanty;* Involuntary and unnoticed; *Corrosive; Offensive, smelling like carrion or the discharge from putrid ulcers* (watery or fluid stools); *Painless (watery stools);* Profuse (brownish-yellow watery stools).

Aggravation: *At night:* **After eating** *or drinking: After midnight: After taking cold: From cold food, ice-water or ice-cream:* From rancid food, *especially spoiled sausage:* During dentition: From milk: From fruit: From acids: During smallpox: During typhoid fever: After abuse of alcohol: After severe external burns: From damp places: At the sea-shore: From motion: In morning after rising.

Amelioration: By external heat (pains).

Before Stool: Chilliness: Anxiety: Cutting in abdomen: Vomiting: Thirst: Feeling as if abdomen would burst: Feeling of constriction in abdomen: Burning in umbilical region: Twisting in abdomen: Coldness in back: Violent screaming: Fainting.

During Stool: Chilliness: Nausea: Vomiting: Colic: Cutting pain: Burning in umbilical region: Cutting pain in anus: *Tenesmus: Burning in anus and rectum:* Sensation of contraction just above the anus: Backache.

After Stool: Relief: *Burning in anus and rectum:* Tremulous weakness, obliging one to lie down: Palpitation of the heart: Perspiration: *Exhaustion:* Prolapsus ani: Eructations.

Accompaniments: **Great restlessness; anguish; constantly changing place.** Child is angry, cross and violent, especially on waking. Child wants to lie with head high. *Fear of death, or of being left alone.* Timorous whimpering. Face pale, earthy, death-like, yellowish. Features distorted and often covered with greenish, cold perspiration. Blue rings around the eyes. Lips black, dry, cracked or blue and cold. Tongue dry, black, or brown, cracked. Aphthæ. Bloody saliva. **Violent, unquenchable, burning thirst, with frequent drinking of small quantities of water.** Desire for acids, cold water or spirits. Loss of appetite. Bitter taste in the mouth after eating or drinking. Nausea at the sight of food. **Vomiting, immediately after eating or drinking;** of food; of drink; of brown or black substances; of blood; of green or yellow-green mucus; of bile; of thick, glassy mucus; with violent pains in the stomach, and *burning in stomach* and abdomen. Abdomen swollen. Urine offensive, scanty, retained, suppressed or greenish. Red and blue spots on the skin. Sleep restless, broken by starts and convulsions. *Stupor with dry, hot skin, twitching of limbs and tonic spasms of the fingers and toes.* The skin is at first hot and dry; later it is icy cold and covered with clammy sweat, although the patient complains of intense burning heat internally; or cold, dry skin may alternate with cold, sticky perspiration.

Great weakness; fainting; rapid exhaustion. *Very rapid and scarcely perceptible pulse*, or the pulse may be fast in the morning and slow in the evening. *Rapid emaciation, with œdema of face and legs.*

There is reason to fear that, as routine is easier than study, **Arsenicum** may have accomplished more harm than good in the hands of homœopathic practitioners. No remedy has been more frequently given in acute affections of the bowels, while it is not the most frequently indicated, and it is not a remedy to be unwisely used. The symptoms which most clearly distinguish it from other remedies with a similar totality are the characteristic thirst and restlessness. These two must be present as a general rule. *The mucous stools are not usually offensive; the watery ones are very much so, and often painless.*

16. ASAFŒTIDA.

Stools: *Yellow; Dark brown;* Greenish; Slimy (only slime passes, no fæces); *Watery;* Papescent; **Disgustingly offensive**; *Profuse.*

Aggravation: After drinking: In hysterical women: In scrofulous children: *At night* (general condition). In syphilitics who have taken much mercury.

Amelioration: By pressure (abdominal symptoms).

Before stool: Colic: Violent urging: Emission of flatus.

During Stool: *Discharge of offensive flatus:* Pain in abdomen.

After Stool: Relief of colic.

Accompaniments: *Hypersensitiveness, either moral or physical.* Ill humor. Irritable mood. Hysterical restlessness and anxiety. Child is clumsy. Greasy taste in mouth, with dryness and burning. *Sensation of a ball rising in the throat, causing dyspnœa. Food, when partially swallowed, returns into the mouth.* Soreness in œsophagus, preceded by burning. Great disgust for all food. Rancid or putrid eructations. *Flatus passes upwards, none downward.* Faint, gone feeling, with strong pulsations in the stomach. Abdominal pulsations. Colic relieved by pressure. Painful distension of abdomen, with *feeling as if peristaltic action were reversed;* relieved by passing flatus. *Constriction of the chest, with dyspnœa.* Twitching and jerking of the muscles. *Hysterical spasms after suppression of habitual discharges, as from an ulcer.* Glands swollen, hard and hot, with shooting, jerking pains.

Asafœtida has a limited range of action, and is

chiefly applicable to diarrhœa occuring in scrofulous children and hysterical women. The extremely offensive stool and generally reversed peristalsis are the leading indications for its use. The general nightly aggravation is important.

17. ASARUM EUROPEUM.

Stools: *Tenacious mucous;* Shaggy masses of mucus, of resinous appearance; Scanty, yellow, stringy mucous; In a long, twisted string; Odorless; Ascarides pass with the stool; Yellowish-brownish; Watery (very weakening); Undigested. Whitish-gray, ash colored, with bloody mucus on top.

Aggravation: In chilly, nervous individuals: From debility: During hectic or slow fever: *In childbed.* After a meal. In cold, dry weather (general).

Amelioration: After vomiting (pain and dulness of head). Cold washing. Damp weather.

Before Stool: Cutting in abdomen: Sharp stitches in the rectum from above downward: Cutting in rectum.

During Stool: Cutting in abdomen and rectum: Nausea: Prolapsus ani.

After Stool: *Prolapsus ani:* Pressing and straining, and discharge of white, viscid, bloody mucus.

Accompaniments: Dulness and pressure in the head. *Cannot bear the sound of scratching on linen or any similar substance.* Food tastes bitter.

Much empty retching, with gurgling and rumbling in the abdomen.

Scanty vomiting of greenish, sour liquid. Loss of appetite or loathing of food. Constantly chilly. Hands, feet, knees or abdomen cold, even in a hot room, or when warmly covered.

The relief from cold bathing and damp weather is very characteristic.

18. ASCLEPIAS TUBEROSA.

Stools: Watery; Black, with yellow spots like fat swimming in them; Yellow; Green; Jelly-like; Like scrapings of the intestines; Offensive; Smelling like rotten eggs; Intense yellow color, with green and yellow flakes; Ascarides with the stool.

Aggravation: At night: After midnight: During the winter: In warm weather, with cold and damp nights: In the autumn.

Before Stool: Colic: Rumbling in the bowels: Violent pain.

During Stool: *Feeling as if a stream of fire passed through the abdomen, and as if bowels would come out:* Tenesmus: Violent colic.

After Stool: Smarting in the rectum: Colic continues: Pain in anus.

Accompaniments: Mental depression. Headache. Flatulent colic. Rheumatic pains in the extremities. Debility, worse after any exertion. Drowsiness, with uneasy sleep and fatiguing dreams.

THEIR INDICATIONS.

The symptoms of **Asclepias** are well-marked and peculiar, but, as yet, lack clinical verification.

19. BAPTISIA TINCTORIA.

Stools: *Consisting of pure blood;* Bloody mucous; Small; Frequent; **Dark, thin fecal**; Papescent, yellowish; Watery; Dark brown mucous and blood; Light yellow, brown, thin and watery; Exhausting; Involuntary; Excoriating; *Horribly offensive; Often painless.*

Aggravation: In hot weather: In the autumn: *During typhoid fever:* Day and night: From solid food.

Before Stool: Colic, more in the hypogastrium: Chills: Pain in limbs and small of back.

During Stool: *Tenesmus:* Colic continues.

After Stool: Tenesmus: Relief of colic.

Accompaniments: Delirious stupor; *falls asleep while answering questions.* **Cannot sleep, head or body feels scattered about the bed; tosses about to get the pieces together. Face dark red, with a besotted look.** Aphthæ, especially in cases of long standing, extending from the mouth through to the anus; sore mouth of nursing infants and consumptives; gums dark, livid, with oozing of blood and fetid odor. **Tongue coated yellowish-brown in the centre, with red, shining edges.** Dry tongue. Little or no thirst. Spits fluid out of mouth or squirts it across the bed. Great sinking at stomach, with frequent fainting. Nausea and vomiting. Nausea with thirst. *Child* *can take nothing but liquids; the slighest amount of solid food causes gagging.* Pain in the region of the liver and particularly of the gall-bladder; worse on walking. Pain and soreness in bowels. *Urine and perspiration extremely offensive. Breath fetid.* Fever slight, pulse soft and full. Sleeplessness, or sleep with heavy, tiresome dreams. *Bruised, sore feeling of the whole body, causing restlessness. Prostration more profound than the severity of the attack would seem to justify.*

Extended clinical observation has proved the value of **Bapt.** in both diarrhœa and dysentery, when assuming the typhoid type. The tenesmus, with absence of pain and the characteristic tongue and mental symptoms, render its selection easy and certain.

20. BARYTA CARBONICA.

Stools: Papescent; Watery; Undigested; Yellow, with mucus and blood; Involuntary.

Aggravation: In scrofulous, dwarfish children: After taking cold: By lying on the painful side (pains).

Before Stool: Sudden urging: Soreness in the lumbar region: Chilliness over the head and legs: Ineffectual urging; Colic.

During Stool: Burning in anus and rectum.

After Stool: Renewed urging: Burning and soreness around the anus.

Accompaniments: *Mental weakness, timidity and imbecility.* Anger with cowardice. *Child* *afraid of strangers; will not play, will not read; prefers to sit idly in a corner; stupid, silly look*. Memory weak. Face flushed. Craving appetite, but feeling of satiety after a few mouthfuls. Aversion to sweets and fruit. Abdomen bloated, while the rest of the body is emaciated. Mesenteric glands enlarged. Sudden irresistible urging to stool, with painful soreness in lumbar region, followed by frequent diarrhœic stools. Pains in small of back. Swelling of cervical glands and tonsils. Rheumatic stiffness and aching of the whole body, in damp weather. Child is slow in learning to walk.

Baryta carb. will occasionally prove useful in the diarrhœa of scrofulous children. The concomitant symptoms and the appearance of the child are more characteristic than the stool.

21. BELLADONNA.

Stools: *Thin, green mucous; Bloody mucous;* Granular, yellow, slimy mucous; White mucous; *White, papescent, fecal (as white as lime);* Clay-colored; Watery; Containing lumps like chalk; Chalky-white, with granular, slimy mucous; Alternating with heat in head; *Small; Frequent; Involuntary* (when passing flatus); Sour smelling (Fetid).

Aggravation: *Afternoon: After sleeping:* After taking cold from cutting the hair: In hot weather: During typhoid fever: From motion: From pressure (colic).

Amelioration: From bending double (colic.)

Before Stool: Perspiration: Heat in the abdomen: Colic: Pinching and contractive griping: Sore aching in upper part of abdomen: Constriction in rectum: *Constant pressing toward the anus and genitals as if everything would be pushed out.*

During Stool: Shuddering: *Tenesmus:* Nausea: Pressing pain in stomach: Pressure on the bladder: Urination: Bearing down pain in uterus: Burning of anus: Perspiration.

After Stool: *Tenesmus:* Shuddering.

Accompaniments: Head hot, while hands and feet are cold. Easily startled. *Rolling the head from side to side.* Delirium; worse during sleep or just after; desire to get out of bed, or into another one. *Stupor. Lethargy*, with pale, cold face, or flushed face, with congested, half-opened, distorted eyes, **dilated pupils,** grating of the teeth, distortion of the mouth, and **violent throbbing of the carotids.** Children cry much and are very cross. Tongue dry, and red at the point and on edges, or has two white stripes on a red ground, or sensation of dryness in mouth, while tongue is moist. Ptyalism. Not much thirst, but desire to moisten the mouth often, or great thirst with desire for cold drinks. Mouth open. Constant chewing. Aversion to food; to meat, beer, acid things. Abdomen distended and tender. Abdomen hot. Sensation of soreness deep in the abdomen; pains more in the left side; aggravated by bending the body to that side. Cutting, tearing, constrictive pains in abdomen, relieved by bending forward. Nausea and vomiting. Belching of wind. Urine profuse or suppressed. Involuntary urination. Several watery stools immediately after profuse sweat: *Partial or general spasms, with unconsciousness, renewed by contact or bright light. Dry heat or hot sweat. Quick hard, small pulse.*

Sleepiness with restlessness; starting up suddenly. Twitching of the muscles during sleep. Moaning during sleep, with half-closed eyes. Drowsiness, with inability to sleep. Every little jar is painful.

The pains appear and disappear suddenly.

Belladonna will be found suitable for children more frequently than adults. It is often the only remedy required for severe cases of infantile dysentery. The drowsiness, with startings, dry heat and frequent drinking, may be regarded as characteristic, if the other symptoms of the patient correspond.

22. BENZOIC ACID.

Stools: *Watery, white, or light-colored;* Like dirty soap-suds; *Copious;* **Very offensive**; Frothy bloody; Smelling strong, pungent, like urine; Putrid, bloody.

Aggravation: In children: During dentition. In gouty, rheumatic, syphilitic or gonorrhœal subjects.

Before Stool: Chilliness: Urging, with ineffectual straining.

During Stool; Urging.

Accompaniments: **Urine very strong smelling; usually dark.** Scanty. Much exhaustion. Weakness. Perspiration. Cold sweat on the head. Sweats while eating.

The symptoms of **Benz. ac.** are not many, but they are genuine jewels. The offensive stools are not like those of any other remedy. The smell is strong, pungent, urinous, somewhat like that of the characteristic urine, which is also almost invariably present.

23. BISMUTHUM.

Stools: Papescent; *Watery; Cadaverous-smelling; Painless.*

Before Stool: Rumbling in the abdomen.

During Stool: Emission of fetid flatus: Colic.

After Stool: Great prostration.

Accompaniments: Desire for company. Pale face, with blue rings around the eyes. *Tongue thickly coated white.* **Thirst: drinks large quantities of water and vomits it immediately.** *Convulsive gagging.* Vomiting occurs as soon as the stomach is full, and is then enormous. **Vomits water only; food is retained.**

Heaviness, pressure and burning in the pit of the stomach.

Abdomen distended with flatulence.

Great prostration, but the surface is warm.

The value of **Bismuth.** in cholera infantum has not been fully appreciated. The excessive prostration, without coldness of the surface, will readily distinguish it from other remedies. In thickly coated white tongue and gastric symptoms it resembles **Antimon. crud.**

24. BOLETUS LARICIS.

(Polyporus officinalis.)

Stools: Yellow, watery; Frothy; Papescent; Mixed with bile and frothy mucus or with oily-looking fluid; Thin, dark, papescent; Mucous; Whitish, mucous; Bilious, mucous and bloody; Bilious, mucous and black fecal; Undigested; Sometimes painless; Profuse; Pouring out in a stream.

Aggravation: In the morning and during the day.

Before Stool: Distress in the hypogastric region.

During Stool: Tenesmus (or absence of pain).

After Stool: Burning pain and distress in the stomach, right lobe of liver, umbilical region and hypogastrium: Terrible distress between stomach and navel: Great faintness and distress in solar plexus: Rumbling in the bowels: Severe tenesmus (or absence of pain).

Accompaniments: Irritable and despondent. Dull frontal headache. Flushed face. Teeth and gums sore. Tongue coated white or yellow, taking the imprints of the teeth. Taste flat, bitter, coppery, or lost. Nausea. Vomiting of sour or bitter fluid. Loss of appetite. Great faintness at the stomach. Dull, aching, dragging or burn-

ing pains in the liver, especially in the right lobe, with burning in the region of the gall-bladder. Pain in the region of the spleen. *Urine thick and high-colored or red and scanty.* Dull, heavy pains in back and legs. Aching in all the joints. Restless after midnight. Very weak and languid. Chilliness along the spine, followed by hot flashes and sweat. Skin hot and dry, especially the palms of the hands. Jaundice.

The value of **Boletus** must be determined by the crucial test of clinical experience. In many of the symptoms it closely resembles **Leptandra**.

25. BORAX.

Stools: *Light yellow, slimy mucous; Green mucous;* Frequent; Yellow watery; Colorless; Fermented; *Thin, brown, frothy,* containing small pieces of yellow fæces; *Offensive, smelling like carrion* (brown stools); *Painless* (brown stools).

Aggravation: *In nursing infants:* During dentition: From fruit (apples, pears): After breakfast: After chocolate: After eating: Afternoon: Evening: In the morning.

Before Stool: Peevish, lazy, dissatisfied: Urging.

During Stool: Burning in the rectum: Faintness and wearines.

After Stool: Cheerful, contented mood.

Accompaniments: *Easily startled at sudden noise.* Apathetic. Crying. **Anxious feeling dur-**

ing downward motion or rocking. Hot head. Pale, clay-colored face. Red eruption on face. Hot mouth. *Aphthæ* on the tongue and inside of the cheek, bleeding when eating. Palate of infants looks wrinkled, *with screaming when nursing*. Loss of appetite (loathing of the breast in infants). Desire for sour drinks.

Vomiting of sour slime (after chocolate).

Constant vomiting, with painless diarrhœa.

Distension by flatulence after every meal.

Pinching in the abdomen. Abdomen soft, flabby and sunken.

Frequent urination, preceded by cries. Urine acrid and fetid.

Starting from sleep with anxious screams, throwing the hands about, seizing things or clinging to the mother. The legs jerk when falling asleep.

Palms hot. Emaciation; flesh relaxed. Skin pale or livid. Debility. Sopor.

Belladonna has, doubtless, been often given when **Borax** should have been. The anxious feeling on downward motion is the chief distinction between them, and is peculiar to **Borax**.

26. BOVISTA.

Stools: Liquid, yellow, fecal; First part hard, last part thin and watery.

Aggravation: *Early in the morning: In the evening:* At night: *Before the menses: During the menses.*

Amelioration: After breakfast.

Before Stool: Urging: Colic.

During Stool: Twisting pains in the abdomen: Cutting pains.

After Stool: Tenesmus: Burning at anus: Languor: Burning and itching in anus as if worms were crawling.

Accompaniments: Nausea in the morning; better after breakfast. Distension of the abdomen, with rumbling shifting of flatulence, and emission of much flatus. Colic which causes the patient to double over, relieved by eating.

Bovista is chiefly useful for diarrhœa, occurring before and during menstruation. The menses are either too early or too late, and the flow is profuse, dark and clotted, occurring mostly at night or early in the morning.

27. BROMINE.

Stools: *Black fecal;* Light yellow, slimy mucous; Painless, *odorless*, like scrapings of the intestines; Yellow, green or blackish.

Aggravation: After a meal: *After oysters*: After acids: At night.

Amelioration: From black coffee: *After eating* (nausea and pains in the stomach).

Before Stool: Cutting and rumbling in abdomen.

During Stool: Much flatus: Pressing in stomach and abdomen: *Blind, intensely painful varices; worse from application of warm and cold water; better after wetting with saliva.*

After Stool: *Blind, intensely painful varices; worse from application of cold and warm water;* better after wetting with saliva.

Accompaniments: Desire for acids. Nausea. Aversion to habitual smoking; it causes nausea and vertigo. Emptiness in the stomach. Contractive spasm of the stomach passing off after eating. Croup of rectum. *Icy coldness of the forearms;* hands cold and moist. Great languor and debility.

One or two cases of **Bromine** diarrhœa, in its characteristic totality, are as many as can be expected to fall to one physician during a lifetime. Should the aggravation after oysters, however, become more fully confirmed, it will need to be used more frequently.

28. BRYONIA.

Stools: Brown, thin fecal; Black; Thin, bloody; Undigested; Green and watery; *Copious, papescent, dark green;* Like dirty water with whitish, finely granulated sediment of undigested food; Painless; Pasty, very offensive; Acrid; Mucus and blood preceded by hard stool; Frequent; Involuntary (during sleep); *Smelling like rotten cheese;* Putrid; Alternating with constipation.

Aggravation: *In the morning*, about 2 or 3 A. M.: *On first rising and moving about: In hot weather: Whenever the weather becomes warmer:* At night: *After suppression of exanthemata;* During typhoid: At the seashore: After taking cold: After cold drinks: After taking milk: From eating stewed fruit or vegetables: From anger or chagrin: After sour kraut: *From sitting up (nausea, etc.):* **From motion, even of a hand or foot:** *From lying on either side.*

Amelioration: *By keeping still: By doubling up or lying on the abdomen* (colic): *By lying on the back.*

Before Stool: Colic: Cutting pains: Nausea: Griping and pinching in abdomen and in region of navel: Constant ineffectual urging.

During Stool: Burning at anus: Prolapsus ani: Vomiting: Thirst: Drowsiness: Chilliness: Offensive flatus: Motion like fermentation in the abdomen: Pain in stomach: Profuse urination.

After Stool: Heat: Drowsiness: Relief.

Accompaniments: Desire for things which do not exist, or which are refused when offered. Peevishness. Ill humor. Delirium. *Desire to get out of bed and go home. Talking of the business of the day. Head hot, with frequent tossing of the hands to the head.* Boring of the head back into the pillows or rolling from side to side. Eyes glassy and staring; sleeps with the eyes half open. Sensitiveness to noise and light. Dry, swollen, cracked lips. *Mouth so dry that the child will not nurse until it is moistened.* Tongue dry and red or brown, or white or yellow. **Thirst for large quantities at long intervals.** *Bitter taste in the mouth, and of food. Nausea and fainting on sitting up.* Much gagging and vomiting. Desire for cold drinks, wine, coffee, sour drinks. Vomiting of bitter substances, of yellow-green mucus. Pain in the bowels after eating or drinking. Urine dark red and clear.

Desire to lie down and remain quiet.

Bryonia has not been one of the routine remedies for loose discharges from the bowels, nor is it desirable that it should become so, or that that list should be enlarged. It is, however, quite often indicated, and, if administered according to the above symptoms, will not fail to repay the careful chooser.

29. CALCAREA CARBONICA.

Stools: Yellowish fecal; Gray, clay-like fecal; *Green;* Chalk-like; Watery; Frothy; *Whitish,* Whitish-gray streaked with blood; Dark greenish brown; Slimy; Creamy; *Large, watery, yellow, merely staining the diaper; Pungent; Fetid; Smelling like rotten eggs; Sour;* Involuntary; *Undigested, containing curdled milk;* Profuse; Frequent; Ascarides with the stool.

Aggravation: *In fat children: In infants with open fontanelles:* In scrofulous persons: In children: *During dentition*: *After milk:* After smoked meat: In summer season: In the afternoon: From sweets: From artificial foods: From bathing (general condition): After eating: After walking and motion.

Before Stool: Great irritability: Nausea.

During Stool: Paleness: Tearing pain in rectum: Prolapsus ani.

After Stool: Faintishness: Lassitude.

Accompaniments: Child is precocious, *obstinate and self-willed*, and cries persistently. Very nervous at night; child cries and has an anxious look when lifted from the cradle. *Head too large, cranial sutures widely open, fontanelles open and sunken*. Scalp thin, showing the veins distinctly. Hair dry, looking like tow. Face sometimes flushed, but usually *pale and bloated*, or *sunken, emaciated, wrinkled and cold*. Pupils dilated. Scrofulous swelling of the upper lip. Gums swollen. Aphthæ. Dry mouth, alternating with salivation. Dentition tardy, and often attended with convulsions and a loose rattling cough. Continued thirst for cold drinks, more at night. Desire for wine, salt or sweet things. Canine hunger in the morning. **Longing for eggs.** Sour taste in the mouth, or of bread. *Sour vomiting or regurgitation, particularly of soured food, milk, etc.* **Pit of stomach swollen like an inverted saucer.** *Swollen, distended abdomen, with emaciation and good appetite.* Enlargement of mesenteric and cervical glands.

Painful and difficult urination, the urine being usually clear, and having a peculiar strong, pungent, fetid odor. Urine is sometimes dark-brown with white sediment. Crawling in the rectum as from worms. Oozing of fluid from the anus, smelling like herring brine. Arms cold to the elbows. *Child does not sleep after 2 or 3 A. M., and is drowsy and weary all day.* Sleep restless with crying out at night; child scratches its head when aroused. Skin either hot and dry, or cold and clammy. Weakness and curvature of spine. Neck too slender to support the head. Curvature of the legs. Ankles weak. Bones weak and bend readily.

Debility. **Profuse sweat on the head when sleeping, especially on the back of the head, wetting the pillow.** *Knees clammy.* **Feet constantly cold and damp.**

In selecting **Calcarea c.**, the stool is of less importance than the person and the concomitant symptoms. These often render it the indispensable remedy in psoric individuals. The smell of the urine cannot be described, but once smelled it is never forgotten. The color will distinguish it from that of **Benz. ac.** It is said to be suitable when persistent tenesmus remains after dysentery in children.

30. CALCAREA PHOSPHORICA.

Stools: *Green, slimy, undigested; Hot, watery;* Purulent; *Spluttering; Extremely offensive;* White; Papescent; Containing pus in small points or flakes; Soft (expulsion difficult); *Expelled forcibly* (green and watery stools); Frequent.

Aggravation: *In scrofulous and rachitic children: During dentition:* From fruit or cider: In the evening: In school girls at puberty: After vexation.

Amelioration: By passing flatus and by lying on the abdomen (abdominal pains).

Before Stool: Cutting, pinching colic.

During Stool: *Emission of much offensive flatus.*

After Stool: Relief of pain in the abdomen: Protruding, aching, sore piles: Renewed urging directly on wiping.

Accompaniments: Peevish and fretful. Intellectual depression and slow comprehension. Head disproportionately large. **Cranial bones (especially occipital) very soft and thin, crackling like paper upon pressure.** *Both fontanelles open*; posterior *fontanelle very large. Sweating of the head. Neck too slender to support the head, which falls from side to side.* Headache, most severe near the sutures, worse after mental exertion and from damp weather. Face pale, sallow, dirty white, brownish, sunken, with blue rings around the eyes. The veins show through the skin. *Nose, chin and tips of ears cold.* Dry mouth and tongue, with much thirst. Teeth develop slowly. *Persistent vomiting of milk. Craving appetite; infant wants to nurse all the time.* **Desire for salted and smoked meats, ham, bacon, etc.** Cold water and ice-cream cause vomiting the next day after taking them. Jellies and sour things cause headache and weakness of the bowels. Crying spells, caused by soreness, aching and colicky pains around the navel, every time the child nurses. Much rumbling of flatus. **Abdomen sunken and flabby.** Mesenteric glands enlarged. Child has anxious expression of the face and suffocative attacks whenever it is lifted from the cradle. Drowsy during the day. Sleep restless, with stretching and yawning. Convulsive starts when lying on the back, ceasing when lying on the side.

Predisposition to glandular swellings and diseases of osseous tissue. Curvature of the spine. Spine so weak in the lumbar region that the child cannot sit upright unless the back is supported. Slow in learning to walk on account of weak ankles.

Rheumatic aching, soreness and stiffness, aggravated by damp weather and by motion.

Great emaciation, the child looking old and wrinkled. Skin dry and cold.

Tendency to marasmus or hydrocephaloid.

Calc. phos. is one of our most valuable remedies for the diarrhœa of scrofulous and rachitic children. It can easily be distinguished from **Calc. c., Silic.,** and **Sul.** by the concomitant symptoms. When given in season it will often prevent marasmus, and is the first remedy to be thought of in threatened hydrocephaloid, after the failure of **China** to arrest the disease.

31. CAMPHOR.

Stools: Dark brown; Blackish; Looking like coffee-grounds (fecal); (Watery?); Large, thin;

Involuntary; Like rice-water; Generally painless; Sour.

Attack very sudden.

Aggravation: During epidemic cholera: From hot sun: After taking cold: In pernicious fevers.

Accompaniments: Great anguish and discouragement. Mental antipathy. Vertigo. *Icy coldness of the whole body*, with chilliness and shaking, or cold, clammy, debilitating perspiration; sometimes occurring only at night, and passing off in the morning. *Coldness of the surface without change of color. Face pale, livid, purple, icy-cold, distorted; upper lip drawn up, exposing the teeth; foam at the mouth; eyes sunken and fixed. Wild, staring, unconscious look.* Aversion to light. *No thirst*, or violent thirst. Nausea and vomiting. Faintness, with pressure at pit of the stomach, and colicky pain. Stomach very sensitive to pressure. Burning in the stomach and œsophagus. *Cramps in the calves.*

Sudden and great sinking of strength. Vomiting and diarrhœa suddenly cease, and the child lies almost unconscious, with blue face and hands, cold tongue, icy coldness of the body, and hoarse, weak voice. Trismus and tetanus.

Stool generally painless.

Cold sweat on the face.

In Cholera: Great sinking and collapse, sometimes without stool or vomiting. **Cold as death, but cannot bear to be covered.**

Camph is principally useful in the very commencement of diseases of the bowels; later stages, presenting similar symptoms, requiring **Verat., Cuprum,** etc. "In **Camph.** collapse is most prominent; in **Verat. alb.** the evacuations and vomiting; in **Cuprum** the cramps."—DUNHAM.

32. CANTHARIS.

Stools: Yellow, brown, watery; **White or pale-reddish mucous stools, like scrapings of the intestines;** *Bloody; Skinny;* Like washings of meat; Bloody mucous; Green mucous; Slimy; Frothy; Frequent; Small; Corrosive.

Aggravation: *At night:* In the evening: During the day: After coffee (pains and loathing): While urinating.

Before Stool: Violent colic: Urging: Pinching in hypogastrium.

During Stool: Colic and pinching continue: Pain in the anus: Pressing and urging, extorting cries: *Burning at the anus:* Prolapse of rectum.

After Stool: Colic relieved, or continues with less violence: *Tenesmus: Burning, biting and stinging in anus:* Shuddering: *Violent chilliness* as though water were poured over one, with internal warmth: Faintness.

Accompaniments: *Anxious restlessness.* Irritability. *Pale, wretched appearance. Deathlike appearance during the pains.* Lips, tongue and palate raw. Vesicles and canker in the mouth and throat. Dryness of the lips. Thirstlessness or violent burning thirst, especially during the pains; but aversion to fluids, because they aggravate the constriction of the throat, the dysuria or the tormina. Aversion to food and to tobacco. Violent pains in abdomen and intestines. Burning in abdomen. Abdomen very sensitive to touch.

Frequent ineffectual desire to urinate, painful. Burning after urination. Hæmaturia. *Retention or suppression of urine, with uræmic coma, delirium and convulsions.*

Collapse, with feeble pulse and cold hands and feet. Burning pains while the surface of the body feels colds.

The appearance like scrapings of the intestines is the most characteristic symptom of **Cantharis**, and will frequently call for it when the more painful and violent symptoms are not present.

33. CAPSICUM.

Stools: *Mucous; Bloody mucous; Tenacious mucous, streaked with black blood; Thin, adhesive, slimy, mixed with black blood; Shaggy, slimy and bloody;* Greenish frothy; *Frequent; Small; Expelled with violence.*

Aggravation: In persons of lax fibre: At night: *After drinking: By currents of air, even warm air (pains).*

Before Stool: Cutting colic: Flatulent colic: Writhing pains about the umbilicus.

During Stool: Cutting and writhing continue: Tenesmus: Burning in lower part of rectum, with sensation of rawness and throbbing and pains in the back: Burning along the sacrum: Strangury: Biting, stinging pain at anus.

After Stool: *Tenesmus: Burning at anus:* **Thirst, drinking causing shuddering**: *Drawing pains in the back.*

Accompaniments: Increased acuteness of all the senses. Homesickness, with redness of cheeks and sleeplessness. Swollen, cracked lips. Flat, watery taste. *Putrid taste, as of putrid water.* Thirstlessness. Food tastes sour. Sour taste in the mouth. Aphthæ, with fetid breath. Desire for coffee, with nausea after taking it. Abdomen much distended. Sensation of coldness in the stomach.

Tenesmus of the bladder, strangury. Frequent, unsuccessful desire to urinate, with burning in the bladder.

Yawning. Sleeplessness.

Capsicum is one of the royal remedies for dysentery; resembling **Canth.** much in its symptoms, but differing equally as much, as a comparison will show. When the choice becomes difficult, the drinking after stool causing shuddering, and the drawing pains in the back after stool, will fix the decision on **Caps.**, and distinguish it also from **Merc. cor.** and **Nux vom.** The patient is also sometimes "lazy, fat, unclean, dreads the open air."

34. CARBO VEGETABILIS.

Stools: Thin, pale mucous; Bloody mucous

(dark, thin fecal); *Brown, watery, slimy;* Light-colored; Semi-liquid, black; Ashy-gray (mushy); Painful; *Frequent; Involuntary* (with flatus); *Putrid; Cadaverous-smelling*.

Aggravation: *After long-continued or severe acute disease:* After loss of fluids: *From chilling the stomach with ice-cream or ice-water, when over heated:* After fat food: After spoiled or rancid food, especially shell-fish: In hot weather: At night: After exposure to great heat of the sun or of fire: In tuberculous patients: In old people.

Before Stool: Slight cutting.

During Stool: Burning and cutting in anus: Tenesmus: Great straining like labor pains to pass a soft stool: *Fetid flatus*.

After Stool: Burning in anus: Trembling weakness: Itching in anus and perineum: Oozing from the rectum.

Accompaniments: *Restlessness and anxiety, worse from 4 to 6 P. M. Child irritable, strikes, bites and kicks. Greenish color, or great paleness of the face*, or cheeks may be red and covered with clammy sweat. The gums recede from the teeth and bleed easily. Desire for coffee. Rancid taste. Flatulent distension of the abdomen, particularly after eating, as though it would burst. Deep-seated burning pains in the abdomen, generally in the bends of the colon. Frequent and violent rancid eructations. *Profuse and constant salivation of stringy saliva. Emission of large quantities of flatus*, inodorous, or *putrid*. Skin pale, or blue and cold. *Feet and legs icy cold to the knees.* Urine offensive or suppressed. Enlarged glands. Emaciation.

In Cholera: *Attack often begins with hæmorrhage from the bowels. Collapse without stool. Nose, cheeks and finger-tips icy cold; lips bluish; cold breath and tongue. Respiration weak and labored.* **Desire to be fanned.** *Cramps in legs and thighs. Hiccough at every motion. Vomiting. Voice hoarse or lost. Pulse thready, intermittent, scarcely perceptible. Consciousness retained or coma.* **Sopor without vomiting, stool or cramps.** Sometimes spasms, followed by congestion of blood to the head or chest.

Except in cholera, **Carbo veg.** is rarely indicated in the beginning of any acute disease of the bowels; but in the later stages it may become the only remedy capable of producing a favorable change. It will not often be required in cases that have had good homœopathic treatment, but much more frequently in those coming from allopathic hands. After it are frequently suitable **Ars., China, Merc. sol.,** or **Psor.** It is also useful for the debility following a long lasting attack of diarrhœa.

35. CARBOLIC ACID.

Stools: Fetid; Rice-water, offensive like rotten eggs; Like thick glue, in thin strips like tape; Bloody and mucous, like scrapings from mucous membrane; Bilious; Watery; Involuntary, thin black stools (in collapse); Involuntary, at night in bed; Diarrhœa alternating with constipation.

Aggravation: From bad drainage: In puerperal fever: In hydrocephalus.

Before Stool: Constant, ineffectual urging.

During Stool: Tenesmus, pain and nausea.

Accompaniments: Patient petulant, impatient. Constantly agitated, moaning continuously and occasionally uttering a piercing cry; delirious starting from sleep. Vomiting. Tenderness over transverse colon. Tongue dry and coated with thick yellow fur. Great thirst and high fever. Urine very dark colored, black or blackish olive green. Vomiting of dark olive green or black fluid, with great restlessness.

"In an exhaustive diarrhœa with very offensive stools, when **Carbo veg.** and **Psorinum** do not help, give **Carbolic acid**."—C. PEARSON.

36. CAUSTICUM.

Stools: Liquid fecal; White mucous; *Possible only while standing;* Involuntary (with flatus).

Aggravation: In the evening: At night: *From cold air striking the abdomen: After eating fresh meat:* In scrofulous children.

Before Stool: Twisting abdominal pains.

During Stool: Vertigo.

After Stool: *Nausea: Salt-water brash:* Vertigo.

Accompaniments: Child cries at the least thing. Afraid of strangers. Timid, fears to go to bed in the dark. Weak memory. Face sallow.

Violently itching acne. Pressure at the pit of the throat, just over the top of the sternum, as of a foreign body, or as of food lodged in œsophagus, causing constant disposition to swallow; better while eating, worse after. *Aversion to sweet things. Fresh meat causes nausea and water brash; smoked meat agrees.* Much thirst for cold drinks. Pressure in the stomach. Necessity to loosen the clothing about the hypochondria. Abdomen swollen and hard; body wasted, and feet disproportionately small. Child walks unsteadily; falls easily.

Involuntary emission of urine, at night; when walking; when coughing.

Causticum will be found useful chiefly in a chronic tendency to diarrhœa, in dyspeptics and consumptives, which is renewed whenever taking fresh meat.

37. CHAMOMILLA.

Stools: *Green slimy mucous; Mixed green and white mucous; Chopped white and yellow mucous;* Green, watery; Yellowish, watery; Changeable; Undigested; Bilious; *Slimy mucous;* Mucous and blood; Like chopped eggs and spinach.

Hot; Small; Frequent; **Smelling like bad eggs;** Sour; Corrosive; Painless (green watery); Painful (thin green slimy); White slimy.

Aggravation: *During dentition: After taking cold:* After anger, chagrin: At night: After tobacco: In childbed: From downward motion: After suppression of perspiration.

Before Stool: Anxiety: *Cutting colic*, worse in epigastric region.

During Stool: *Colic:* Eructations: Nausea: Retching: Thirst: Vertigo: Perspiration, with anxiety: Burning in anus: Violent colic, forcing screams.

After Stool: Relief: Stitches in rectum: Soreness of the anus.

Accompaniments: Desire for many things which are rejected when offered. *Peevishness. Ill humor.* Moaning on account of trifling offense, or because refused what he wants. Whining restlessness; child wants this or that, which, when offered, is refused or pushed away. **Children cry much, and are only stilled by being carried about**. Rheumatic pains in the head. *Redness of the cheeks, or of one cheek only*. Red rash on the cheeks. Gums hot and swollen. Tongue and mouth dry. Tongue coated thick yellow, or white. Bitter, sour, or slimy taste. Aversion to food. Intense thirst. Bitter eructations. Sour vomiting of food or slimy mucus. Abdomen hard and distended. Weight and burning in the stomach. Cutting or tearing colic, making the child bend double and draw up its knees. Involuntary emission of urine which feels hot.

Very painful cutting jerks from right shoulder toward head, with thirst and debility.

Moaning in the sleep, with *hot, sticky sweat on*

forehead. Twitching of the muscles during sleep.

Convulsions: Both legs moved up and down alternately: Grasping with the hands: Mouth drawn to and fro: Eyes staring: Eyes and face distorted: Stupor: Cough, with rattling in the chest: Yawning and stretching.

Novices often fail with **Chamomilla**. It is not adapted to every case of diarrhœa during dentition. The mental symptoms are of chief importance (compare **Cina**), but the desire to be carried about is not alone decisive. If, however, the other symptoms correspond, particularly of the stool, this symptom will make the choice more certain. **Cham.** is not often indicated in cases of long continuance, and is often unable to complete the cure alone, requiring to be followed by **Merc. sol.** or **Sulph.**

38. CHELIDONIUM MAJUS.

Stools: *Thin, bright yellow, fecal;* Brown watery; White watery; Mucous; Pasty, light-gray; Fluid, often involuntary; Painless; Green mucous; Like rice-water tinged yellow; Pale slimy; Yellow watery, containing flakes of mucus; Slimy, grayish-green; Flakes, strings, gelatinous lumps; Alternation of constipation and diarrhœa; Deficiency of biliary coloring matter.

Aggravation: At night (white watery, mucous); From affection of liver.

Amelioration: From wine (colic): From hot drinks.

Before Stool: Rumbling in the abdomen: Nausea.

During Stool: Rumbling in abdomen: Nausea.

After Stool: Rumbling in abdomen.

Accompaniments: Depression of spirits. Sadness. Slimy, white-coated tongue. Disgusting or bitter taste, food tasting natural. Metallic acid taste. Diminished appetite. Desire for wine; *for milk, which agrees; for hot drinks, which agree. Aversion to cheese and boiled meat.* Pain in the stomach, relieved by eating. *Jaundice.* Urine profuse, pale, reddish, yellow or green. **Constant pain under the inferior angle of the right scapula.**

Drowsiness, with inability to sleep.

The **Chelidonium** combination of symptoms is not very common. Clinical experience with it is therefore meagre. The desire for hot drinks is very peculiar, and may prove characteristic.

39. CHINA.

Stools: *Yellow, watery; Undigested;* Blackish; Brownish, thin watery; Chocolate colored; Black, watery; Bilious; Whitish; Greenish; Bloody; Yellow mucous; *Profuse; Frothy;* Frequent; *Involuntary; Putrid; Cadaverous;* Corrosive; *Painless* (undigested and watery stools).

Aggravation: **After a meal: At night:** Early in the morning: In hot weather: In inveterate drunkards: In nursing women: *From fruit:* From drinking sour beer: After measles: During small-

THEIR INDICATIONS. 79

pox: *After severe acute disease: After loss of fluids:* On alternate days: *Afternoon (colic).*

Amelioration: By bending double (colic).

Before Stool: Colic.

During Stool: Stitches and acrid feeling in anus: Thirst: Passage of flatus.

After Stool: Tingling in the rectum, as from worms: Feeling of great debility: Colic.

Accompaniments: Indifference. Vertigo, with sensation as if sinking through the bed. Pale, earthy, bloated face. Lips dry, black, chapped. Ptyalism. Tongue coated white or yellow. Diminished appetite. Voracious appetite, worse at night. Bitter or sour taste. Bitter taste of all kinds of nourishment. Desire for sour things; wine; fruit; cherries. *Desire to drink frequently, but little at a time.* Vomiting of food, of water, of sour mucus, of bile. Enlargement of the liver and spleen. Colic, often violent, of pinching character, with nausea, with thirst, relieved by bending double, *returning every afternoon.* Cutting about the umbilicus, with cold sweat on the forehead. *Distension of the abdomen, temporarily relieved by belching. Fermentation in the bowels. Tympanitis. Emission of large quantities of flatulence,* sometimes very fetid.

Dark urine.

Pulse hard, rapid, irregular.

Great weakness, particularly with the painless

stools. *Inclination to sweat. Profuse night sweats.* Sleep worse after 3 A. M.

Rapid exhaustion and emaciation.

After a long-lasting attack of cholera infantum child becomes drowsy, pupils dilated, rapid and superficial breathing; chin, nose and tips of the ears cold (impending hydrocephaloid).

During Convalescence: Much weakness and debility, with pale *face, ringing in the ears* and tendency to dropsical swelling.

China has a very strong resemblance to **Carbo veg.** The character of the stool will usually serve to distinguish them, together with the fact that with the former the stools are often entirely in the night, being absent during the day, even in severe cases, unless they occur after meals, which is also an additional distinction. When well selected **Chin.** usually completes the cure. In threatened hydrocephaloid, however, it is often necessary to follow with **Calc. phos.**

40. CICUTA VIROSA.

Stool: *Thin, slimy;* Black offensive; Frequent, liquid; *Expelled suddenly.*

Aggravation: At 2 and 5 A. M.: By pressure (abdominal pains).

Before Stool: *Sudden urging, scarcely able to retain the stool;* Burning pain in the back: Weakness.

During Stool: *Violent urging to urinate.*

After Stool: Prolapsus recti: Burning in the anus: Urging: *Desire to urinate*.

Accompaniments: Anxiety and fretfulness. Headache. Vertigo. Pupils dilated. Face pale or flushed. Dryness of the throat, with thirst. *Great longing for charcoal.* Nausea in the morning and when eating. Loss of appetite after eating a few mouthfuls. Burning, swelling and throbbing in the pit of the stomach. Abdomen distended with flatulence. Frequent emission of flatus. Tearing pains deep in the abdomen. Sudden, sharp, stitching pains from the navel to the neck of the bladder. Bruised feeling of the fore-arms and legs. *Frequent involuntary jerking of the arms and fingers*, with sticking pains. Cold extremities. *Frequent waking with sweat all over; feels invigorated.* Chilliness.

In Cholera: *Loud sounding, dangerous hiccough.* Vomiting alternates with *violent tonic spasms of the pectoral muscles*. Congestion of blood to the brain or chest after vomiting ceases. *Violent jerking backward of the head.* Staring or upturned eyes. Heavy breathing. Sopor. Convulsions.

Cicuta is reported to have been used successfully in cholera, but clinical experience with it in diarrhœa is very meagre. The early morning stool, with its peculiar concomitants, the distended abdomen, and the longing for charcoal, seem to furnish characteristic indications.

41. CINA.

Stools: Greenish, slimy; Bilious; **White, mucous, like little pieces of popped corn;** *Reddish mucous;* Bloody; Alternating with constipation; Involuntary; Frequent; Watery.

Aggravation: *During dentition:* In the daytime: After drinking: In children.

Before Stool: Pinching colic.

During Stool: Discharge of round worms.

Accompaniments: Disposed to cry much. Cross and peevish. Rejects everything that is offered. Paleness of the face, *particularly around the nose and mouth*, and sickly appearance around the eyes. *Disposition to pick or bore in the nose.* Grinding of the teeth during sleep. Appetite capricious or impaired. Cutting and pinching in abdomen.

White, turbid urine. White, jelly-like urine. Restless sleep; waking frequently, or frequently changing position, waking with cries. Will not sleep without rocking. Grinding of the teeth during sleep. Worm spasms: the child stiffens out straight.

The accompanying symptoms, particularly those italicized, will more frequently indicate **Cina** than the character of the stools, and will render the choice easy. The characteristic urine is the surest indication.

42. CISTUS CANADENSIS.

Stools: Thin, grayish-yellow, fecal.

Hot; Squirting out.

Aggravation: After-part of the night till noon: After eating: *After fruit: After coffee:* In wet weather (general condition): In scrawny, scrofulous children.

Before stool: *Irresistible urging*.

Accompaniments: Characteristic sore throat. Much dryness of the throat, worse after sleeping, better after eating and drinking. Throat looks glassy. On back of throat stripes of tough mucus. Desire for cheese, for acid food and fruit. Nausea. Pain in the stomach after eating. Cervical glands swollen or suppurating. Goitre.

The irresistible urging to stool early in the morning is like **Sulph.**, but the color and consistence of the stool are different.

43. COCCULUS.

Stools: Yellow, soft, fecal; Slimy; Fetid; Frequent; Painless; Watery; Thin; Black slimy, very fetid.

Aggravation: Directly after rising: From standing: From riding but a short distance in omnibus or car: During intermittent fever: After drinking cold water: Through the day: When bending double (pains).

Amelioration: By sitting: By suppressing the stool.

Before Stool: Urging: Burning in rectum Emission of hot flatus.

During Stool: Pain in bowels, causing dyspnœa, sweat and faintness: Burning in rectum: Vomiting: Flatus.

After Stool: Violent tenesmus: Fainting: Prolapsus recti.

Accompaniments: Metallic, coppery taste in the mouth. Sourish taste after a meal. Intense thirst while eating. Aversion to food; tobacco; drinks; acids. Food tastes as though salted too little. Nausea, with tendency to faint. *Excessive nausea and vomiting when riding in a carriage, or when becoming cold.* Violent spasm of the stomach, with griping, tearing pains. Much rumbling in the bowels. Pain in left side of the abdomen, aggravated when bending double. Sensation of sharp stones rubbing together in abdomen.

Numb, paralytic sensation of the legs.

Fetid, or hot flatus. Watery urine.

Hectic fever. Emaciation.

44. COFFEA.

Stools: Liquid, fecal; Watery; Painless; Offensive; Weakening; Alternation of constipation and diarrhœa.

Aggravation: During dentition: In infants: *From sudden joy:* From taking cold: In open air: From domestic cares: After abuse of chamomile: In old people.

Accompaniments: Over-sensitiveness. *Excitement. Wakefulness.* Colic, as if the stomach had been overloaded. Aversion to open air, which also aggravates the symptoms.

45. COLCHICUM.

Stools: *Watery;* Changeable, greenish, yellowish, reddish, slimy, fecal; *Jelly-like mucous; White, jelly-like mucous, with spots and streaks of blood;* Transparent, mucous; *Bloody, mingled with a skinny substance; White mucous;* Orange-yellow, watery, with bright yellow flakes; Watery, containing *large quantities of white shreddy particles;* mixed with small white membranes or light bluish matter.

Profuse; Frequent (watery); Small; Frequent (bloody and mucous); Painless (watery); Slimy; Offensive; Involuntary and without sensation to the patient (watery); Excoriating; Slightly sour-smelling.

Aggravation: *In the autumn:* In hot, damp weather: In the evening and night: In rheumatism:

From motion (vomiting).

Before Stool: *Griping colic, must bend double:* Constant ineffectual urging: Flatulency: Pinching in abdomen.

During Stool: Borborygmus: Cutting colic: Deathly nausea and prostration: Vomiting, faintness: Pain in anus: *Violent tenesmus: Prolapsus ani:* Spasms of sphincter ani: Shuddering over the back: Pain in small of back.

After Stool: *Tenesmus:* Relief of colic: Long-lasting, agonizing pains in rectum and anus: *Exhaustion: Child falls asleep on the vessel as soon as the tenesmus ceases.*

Accompaniments: *Peevish;* external impressions, light, noise, strong smells, contact, etc., disturb the temper. *Paleness.* Heat in the mouth, with thirst. *Great thirst,* even burning, unquenchable. *Increased secretion of saliva, often very profuse.* The saliva causes nausea and inclination to vomit when swallowing it. Constriction of the œsophagus. Aversion to food on looking at it, *and particularly when smelling of it.* **The smell of fish, eggs, fat meats or broth causes nausea even to faintness.** Violent vomiting occurring with great ease (with the watery stools). Vomiting of yellowish mucus, very bitter prereded by long and violent gagging Every motion excites or renews the vomiting.

Burning in the stomach or icy coldness, also in the abdomen. Colic. Distension of the abdomen, with flatulence. Great swelling of the lower part of the abdomen. Coldness and œdema of the legs; cramps in the calves. Ascites. Urine dark brown and scanty.

Much weakness and prostration.

Colch. stands next to **Podoph.** in painless cholera morbus. It differs chiefly in the stools being smaller and less gushing; in the time of aggravation, and the presence of the nausea and vomiting.

In dysentery the jelly-like and skinny stools are quite characteristic, particularly the latter.

THEIR INDICATIONS. 87

Other symptoms distinguish it from **Aloe.**, **Canth.** and **Kali bich.**

46. COLOCYNTHIS.

Stools: Brownish-yellow fecal; *Saffron yellow, frothy, liquid; First watery and mucous, then bilious, and lastly bloody; Bloody; Bilious;* Slimy and bloody like scrapings of the intestines; *Thin, greenish, slimy and watery;* Thin mucous (painless); Undigested; Increasingly colorless and watery;

Excoriating; Frequent; Not profuse;

Sour putrid; Musty, like brown paper burning.

Aggravation: From cold diet: From sour things: *From eating or drinking: After a meal: From fruit:* From motion: *After vexation, indignation, or grief from ill-treatment: During dentition:* During nursing or right after.

Amelioration: From coffee: Smoking: Pressure: Lying on the abdomen: *Bending double:* By violent exercise (pains): From getting warm in bed.

Before Stool: Difficulty of retaining the stool: *Cutting colic: Great urging:*

During Stool: Tensive pain in the forehead: Cutting colic: Tenesmus: Nausea: Burning along the urethra: Burning in anus: Violent pains in bowels, extending down thighs: Compressive, griping pains, beginning at navel and passing down to rectum: Much flatus.

After Stool: Cessation of colic (or, more rarely,

the colic occurs chiefly, and is very severe after stool): *Weakness, paleness and great prostration:*

Burning and darting pains in the anus: Severe burning along the sacrum.

Accompaniments: Tongue coated white or yellow. Tongue feels scalded. Burning at the tip of the tongue. Bitter taste in the mouth. Canine hunger. Much thirst. Nausea, with fruitless efforts to vomit, lasting until falling asleep, and returning on awaking. Vomiting of food without nausea. Vomiting of bile; of greenish substances.

Intense griping, cutting or squeezing in the intestines, coming up into the stomach and causing nausea, or extending down into the thighs. Squeezing as though between stones. Cutting, lancinating pains flying all over the abdomen. *Pains are aggravated by eating or drinking.* Abdomen feels empty and sore. Tympanitic distension of the abdomen. Rumbling in abdomen. Urine fetid, viscid, jelly-like. Frequent urging to urinate, with small discharge. Retention of urine. Cramps in the legs and feet. Warm feet with cold hands. Chills proceeding from the abdomen.

Sleeplessness.

The characteristic pains of **Coloc.** remain always its prominent indication. Whether they occur before or after stool, or during the interval, it will remove them, and with them, usually, the whole train of symptoms. Sometimes in dysentery, with much tenesmus, **Merc.** is needed afterward.

47. COLOSTRUM.

Stools: *Green, watery; Yellow; Watery;* Mucous; Bilious; *Profuse; Sour-smelling;* Excoriating.

Aggravation: *In nursing infants. During dentition.*

During Stool: Colicky pains in the hypogastrium.

Accompaniments: Great nervous irritability or listlessness.

Pale face. Tongue coated white or yellow.

Vomiting of sour or bitter substances.

Loss of appetite.

The whole body smells sour.

Fever. Emaciation.

The symptoms of **Colostrum** are purely clinical, and like those of all other remedies, which claim recognition solely upon the basis of empiricism, must be regarded with distrust. Only a careful proving and more extended clinical observation can determine their real value.

48. CONIUM.

Stools: *Liquid fecal, mingled with hard lumps; Watery; Undigested;* Sour;

Frequent; Involuntary (during sleep without waking); Alternate constipation and diarrhœa.

Aggravation: During the day.

Before Stool: Cutting pains.

During Stool: Chilliness: Tenesmus: Burning in the rectum.

After Stool: Palpitation of the heart, sometimes intermittent: Tremulous weakness, passing off in the open air, or when lying: Faintness.

Accompaniments: Face pale or sallow. Much vertigo when lying down, and especially when turning over in bed. Desire for acids: salt food; coffee. Nausea after eating. Much inflation of the abdomen after meals, particularly after milk. Emission of fetid or cold flatus.

Cuttings and gripings in the abdomen. *Frequent urination. Intermittent stream of urine; the flow stops and starts repeatedly.* Yellow color of the skin. Jaundice.

Much weakness and lassitude, with desire to sit or lie.

In chronic diarrhœa of old men **Con.** is sometimes the remedy, as indicated by the stool and the urinary symptoms, with the tremulous weakness. It may also become indicated by the same symptoms in younger persons, and then, usually, women.

49. COPAIVÆ.

Stools: *White* fecal; Bloody; Watery;

Copious; Involuntary; Greenish, mixed with mucous flocculi; White mucous in masses; Diarrhœa alternating with obstinate constipation.

Aggravation: In the morning: After taking cold: With bronchial and intestinal catarrh.

Amelioration: By bending double (colic).

During Stool: Drawing, tearing colic: Chilliness: Tenesmus: Nausea and vomiting.

Accompaniments: Loss of appetite. Nausea. Vomiting.

The most characteristic thing of **Copaivæ** is a tendency to a general catarrhal condition and aggravation from taking cold; in both of which it resembles **Dulcamara**.

50. CORNUS CIRCINATA.

Stools: *Dark, bilious, greenish, slimy;* Watery; Mucous;

Very offensive; Frequent and scanty.

Aggravation: After eating: In the morning: During dentition: In jaundice: In liver derangement.

Amelioration: By passage of offensive flatus.

Before Stool: Urging: Colic.

During Stool: Griping pains about the umbilicus: Rumbling and passage of much very offensive flatus: Burning in rectum and anus: Tenesmus: Nausea: Drowsiness, dulness of head and general perspiration.

After Stool: Burning in rectum and anus: Relief of dulness in the head, and distension of stomach: Colic.

Accompaniments: Entirely indisposed to

mental or physical exertion. Cannot think or read. Great relaxation of mind and body.

Dulness and weight in the head, particularly the temples, relieved by coffee. Dark rings around the eyes. Conjunctiva yellow. *Yellow color of the face Face hollow, with an expression of weakness and dulness.* Heat in the face without redness. Tongue coated white or yellow. Aphthæ. Bitter taste. Thirst for cold drinks. Nausea, with general sticky sweat and feeling of exhaustion. Pain in the stomach after eating, with distension of the stomach and abdomen, better after passage of flatus and stool.

Rattling and rumbling in abdomen. Griping pains.

Weakness of the extremities. Sleepiness. Chilliness, followed by flashes of heat and sweat. Debility.

Cornus c. deserves more attention, and will be found frequently useful by those who make the most of every well-proved remedy.

Compare with **Chelid.**

50. CROTALUS HORRIDUS.

Stools: Liquid dark green; Yellow watery; Black, thin; Dark fluid, bloody; Involuntary (dark bloody); Offensive.

Aggravation: From noxious effluvia; From imbibation of septic matter in food or drink; From "high game;" In summer; In low septic states.

During Stool: Colic, nausea, great debility and faintness: Vomiting and micturition simultaneously.

After Stool: Great debility.

Accompaniments: Lowness of spirits and indifference to everything. Disagreeable sensation through the whole body and nauseous taste. Sudden and extreme coldness and blueness.

Collapse, cramps, vomiting.

Embarrassment of respiration.

Scarcely perceptible pulse. Suppression of urine.

Crotalus is one of our most valuable remedies in the most dangerous cases, such as bilious remittents, yellow fever, pyæmia, hectic fever, typhus, relapsing fever; when the diarrhœa takes on the characteristics of the remedy.

52. CROTON TIGLIUM.

Stools: **Yellow watery**; Dark green, or greenish-yellow liquid; Tenacious mucous; *Brownish-green; Undigested;*

Frequent; Small (mucous stools);

Profuse (yellow, watery stools);

Coming out like a shot.

Aggravation: **After drinking**: **While nursing**: **While eating**: At every movement: From fruit: From sweetmeats: During the day: During the summer.

Amelioration: From hot milk (colic): After sleeping.

Before Stool: Heat: Anxiety: Cutting pain in the bowels.

During Stool: Sweat: Nausea: Colic: Cutting in abdomen: Faint feeling: Vomiting: Tenesmus: Scraping of posterior wall of rectum: Disagreeable sensation through the whole body: Nauseous taste: Protrusion of the rectum.

After Stool: Sweat on the forehead: Vertigo: Face sunken and altered in expression: Rumbling and gurgling in left side of abdomen: Burning in anus: Pressing in epigastrium and umbilicus, with protrusion of rectum and constant urging to stool: Nausea, with fainting: *Great pallor and weakness:* Coldness of body.

Accompaniments: Dry, parched lips. Excessive nausea, with vanishing of sight. Gagging, with vertigo, worse after drinking. Vomiting immediately after drinking. Violent vomiting of ingesta; of yellowish-white frothy fluids. Burning and pressure in the stomach. Colic and writhing around the umbilicus. On pressing on the umbilicus with the hand, a painful sensation is felt all along the intestinal canal to the termination of the rectum, causing the latter to protrude somewhat.

The three highly characteristic symptoms of **Crot. tig.**, the yellow watery stool, sudden expulsion and aggravation from drink and food, form a trio whose presence will render success certain and brilliant. This stool is not always

THEIR INDICATIONS. 95

painful. The other stools have the same conditions and are also quickly cured by this remedy.

53. CUBEBÆ.

Stools: Blackish, yellowish, fecal; *Yellow, transparent, mucous; mingled mith whitish shining particles looking like kernels of rice;* Bloody mucous;

Frequent (dysenteric stool); Copious (bilious and fecal); Involuntary.

Aggravation: At night, in bed (colic): From food or drink.

Amelioration: From rising from the bed and moving about (colic).

Before Stool: Cutting pains in hypogastrium: Severe griping pain in bowels, with backache.

During Stool: Headache and griping: Severe griping pains in bowels, with backache: Urging to urinate: Rumbling and cutting in abdomen: Burning in rectum: Tenesmus: Cutting pains: Loud discharge of flatus.

After Stool: Long-continued tenesmus and relief of pains, except dull heavy pain in back and bowels.

Accompaniments: Desire for delicacies; oranges; acid fruits; spirits; brandy; fresh bread; onions; almonds; nuts. Unquenchable thirst, with feeling of dryness of the mouth, though moistened with an oily saliva. Nausea. Abdomen distended and very sensitive.

54. CUPRUM MET.

Stools: Watery; With flakes; Bloody; Black, watery; Green; *Frequent;* Not very copious.

Aggravation: During epidemic cholera: In pernicious intermittents.

Amelioration: From drinking cold water (vomiting).

Accompaniments: *Restlessness, tossing about and constant uneasiness.* Changed features, full of anguish. Spasmodic distortion of the face. Face and lips blue and cold. *Sunken, deep eyes, with blue rings around them.* Excessive thirst. Sweet taste in the mouth. Sweet, stringy saliva. Tip of the tongue cold. All food tastes like clear water. *Desire for warm food and drinks.* Drink descends the œsophagus with a gurgling sound.

Deathly nausea. Violent vomiting; of bile; of water containing flakes, *with violent colic and cramps.* Violent pains in the stomach. Hardness of the abdomen, with extreme sensitiveness to touch. Downward pressure in the hypogastrium. *Spasm of the stomach. Deathly feeling of constriction beneath the sternum. Violent spasms in the abdomen and upper and lower limbs, with piercing screams. Spasms of the throat preventing speech. Dyspnœa so intense that he cannot bear a handkerchief before the face.* Sighing respiration.

Urine scanty and seldom, or suppressed.

Violent cramps in the legs and feet.

Soft, slow pulse, weak and small.

Comatose sleep after vomiting. *Intense coldness and blueness of the surface, with long-continued general cold sweat and great prostration.*

General convulsions, with continued vomiting and violent colic. Uræmic eclampsia with loquacious delirium, followed by apathy, cold tongue and breath, and collapse. **Spasms, with blue face and thumbs clenched across the palms of the hands.**

The violent cramps and spasms of **Cuprum** will distinguish it from **Camph.**, **Verat.** and **Arg. nit.** These cramps particularly affect the flexors, the muscles often drawing up into visible knots.

55. CYCLAMEN.

Stools: Yellow, watery; Papescent; Mucus; Expelled forcibly.

Aggravation: *After coffee:* After pork and fat food: In the evening, during rest, and *in the open air* (general condition).

Before Stool: Pinching colic: Urging: Nausea.

During Stool: Tenesmus: Burning in anus: Colic: Palpitation.

After Stool: Ineffectual straining: Pinching in abdomen: Dulness and forgetfulness.

Accompaniments: Despondency, listlessness. Semi-lateral headache, worse in the left temple, with heat in the head, and almost complete obscuration of sight; relieved by application of cold water. Vertigo, worse in the open air. Pupils dilated or alternately contracted and dilated. Face pale, with blue rings around the eyes. Partial loss of taste or bitter taste. Salivation. Tongue coated white, with red tip; vesicles on the tongue. Aversion to fat food; to bread. Desire for lemonade. Much thirst or absence of thirst. Eructations. Nausea. Vomiting of mucus. Feeling of satiety after a few mouthfuls of food. Pressure and distension in the stomach and abdomen. Rumbling of flatus. Hypogastrium sensitive to pressure. Palpitation of the heart. Sleep restless, disturbed by vivid dreams; falls asleep late and awakens early, with feeling of great lassitude and weakness. Pulse feeble. *Chlorosis*.

In many of its symptoms **Cyclamen** is almost identical with **Puls.**, but may be distinguished from the latter by the character of the stool, the aggravation after coffee and the aversion to open air. Like **Puls.**, it will prove especially valuable for the diarrhœa of chlorotic women, subject to sick headaches and menstrual irregularities.

56. DIGITALIS.

Stools: Watery, fecal and mucous; Yellowish-white fecal; *Whitish, or ash-gray fecal;* Involuntary; Like coffee gounds.

Aggravation: *During jaundice:* Afternoon, five to six o'clock (vomiting).

Before Stool: Cutting or tearing colic: Chilliness: Fainting: Vomiting.

During Stool: Cutting and tearing pains in abdomen.

After Stool: Urging in the rectum: Faintness.

Accompaniments: Pale face, with bluish hue under the pale skin.

Yellow color of face and conjunctiva. Tongue coated white. Mouth, tongue and gums sore. *Fetid or sweetish ptyalism.* Loss of appetite, with clean tongue. Thirst, with desire for sour drinks. Desire for bitter food. Violent nausea, with anguish and great despondency. *Violent vomiting of food; of green bile; of mucus.* Vomiting is sometimes accompanied by external heat, mingled with chills, and followed by perspiration with chilliness. The nausea is not relieved by vomiting.

Tenderness of the liver.

Constant desire to urinate, only a small quantity being passed each time. Great weakness. *Feeling of sinking at the stomach, as though one would die.* **Weak, slow pulse.**

Violent beating of the heart, not rapid, but too violent.

Chest and bowel symptoms alternate; cough in one fit of sickness and diarrhœa in the next.

Digitalis is chiefly indicated by white stool, with symptoms of jaundice and the sinking at the stomach.

57. DIOSCOREA VILLOSA.

Stools: Deep yellow, thin, fecal; Bilious; Watery; Albuminous; Lumpy;

Profuse; Hot; Offensive; White, slimy, jelly-like; Alternate constipation and diarrhœa (during pregnancy).

Aggravation: By sitting, or *lying, or bending double (colic):* In the morning, driving one out of bed.

Amelioration: By eating· In open air (nausea and general symptoms): By currant-wine, pressure and *walking (colic).*

Before Stool: *Colic:* Urging: Drawing pains in the sacrum.

During Stool: *Severe* tenesmus: Burning in the rectum: Emission of much offensive flatus.

After Stool: Hæmorrhoids: Weak, faint feeling in abdomen: The colic continues.

Accompaniments: Nausea. Vomiting. Eructations. **Violent twisting colic, occurring in regular paroxysms, with remissions.** *Severe, drawing, writhing pains in sacral region and bowels, radiating upward and downward, until the whole body and even the fingers and toes become involved in spasms, so severe as to elicit shrieks.*

Abdominal pains suddenly shift and appear in distant localities, as the fingers or toes.

Pains in the legs and knees, relieved by motion and by rubbing.

Disposition to paronychia.

Diosc. has a much narrower range thar **Coloc.**, but, as in the latter, the colic is the principal indication. It is easily distinguished from the colic of any other remedy by the above symptoms. The disposition to felons may be found with the tendency to colic. Whether met with thus or single, **Diosc.** will usually cure whitlow if taken as soon as the pricking in the finger is felt, and greatly relieve and hasten the termination if taken later.

58. DULCAMARA.

Stools: *Yellowish, greenish, watery; Whitish, watery, with flocculi;* White, mucous; *Green, mucous;* Yellow, mucous; *Slimy mucous; Bloody;* Bilious; *Changeable;* Expelled with much force; Dark brown fecal; Involuntary; Undigested;

Sour smelling;

Frequent; Scanty; Corrosive.

Aggravation: *After taking cold: When the weather becomes colder: In the summer when the days are hot and the nights cold and damp:* During wet and cold weather: *At night:* During dentition: After cold drinks: After ice-cream: In the afternoon: In childbed: During pregnancy: In the evening: From going into damp places.

Before Stool: Perspiration: Nausea: Griping colic: Cutting in abdomen.

During Stool: Colic: Perspiration: Heat: Thirst: Eructations: Vomiting: Prolapse of rectum: Faintness.

After Stool: Thirst: Relief, but feeling of weakness: Burning at anus: Tenesmus.

Accompaniments: Impatience. Languor or restlessness. Pale face. Aphthæ. Dry tongue. Spongy gums, with ptyalism of tenacious, soap-like saliva. Much thirst for cold drinks. Loss of appetite. Nausea. Vomiting of mucus; of tenacious mucus. Pinching and cutting colic. *Dry heat of the skin. General prostration.*

Dulc. is seldom required except in cases directly traceable to taking cold or to a change in the weather from warm to cold; but then it becomes the indispensable and often all-sufficient remedy, whether the attack is diarrhœa or dysentery. It is rarely useful if the attack is painless. In many symptoms it resembles **Acon.** and **Arsen.**

59. ELATERIUM.

Stools: *Frothy, watery;* Dull, olive-green discharges; Bilious; Squirting out; Dark green mucous stool, in masses mixed with whitish mucus streaked with blood;

Very frequent and copious (watery); Frequent (mucous).

Aggravation: After taking cold by standing on damp ground after exertion.

Before Stool: Constant urging: Great pain in abdomen.

During Stool: Cutting pain in abdomen: Vomiting.

Accompaniments: Bitter taste. Nausea. Vomiting of watery, greenish, bilious matter, with great weakness.

Oppression, stricture and pain in the epigastrium, with difficult breathing. Violent cutting pains in the abdomen. Chilliness, with continued yawning. Great prostration. Violent flatulent colic following an obstinate diarrhœa.

60. FERRUM METALLICUM.

Stools: Watery; Slimy, mucous; *Undigested;* Corrosive; Involuntary; *Painless;* Sudden, gushing; Brown; Like rice-water; Flaky mucous; Look like intestinal scrapings; Slimy, bloody; Odorless; Exhausting.

Aggravation: After abuse of Cinchona: **While eating or drinking**: *At night:* Mornings: During pregnancy: From least motion: Regularly every afternoon: In phthisical subjects.

Before Stool: Rarely pain.

During Stool: Prolapsus recti (in children): Tenesmus: Burning at anus.

After Stool: Cramping pain in rectum: Burning at anus.

Accompaniments: Rush of blood to the head. Flushed face. Pale face, with red spot on each cheek. **Face flushes easily on the least excitement or exertion.** Canine hunger, alternating with loss of appetite. Aversion to acids, ale, eggs, meats, which also disagree, particularly meats. Unquenchable thirst, or thirstlessness. Vomiting of food soon after eating; of sour and acrid substances. Feeling of weight in abdominal viscera, as though they would fall down when walking. Abdomen feels sore and bruised to the touch, and when walking. Hard and distended abdomen, without flatulence. Spasmodic pain in back and anus. Peevish, tearful. *Emaciation. Debility. Chlorosis.* Exhausting sweats. Coldness of surface, with sour sweat. Failing pulse. Vox choleraica.

Ferrum is sometimes required in cases of chronic diarrhœa, in both adults and children, with the above symptoms. Were it not for its excessive abuse by the allopathists, from whom such cases mostly come, it would be more frequently useful. It must also be remembered in cholera and cholerine; especially when the slightest attempt at eating, drinking or moving brings on a stool.

61. FLUORIC ACID.

Stools: Watery; Yellowish-brown, fecal; Offensive; Very loose, bright yellow, with mucus; Frothy mucus; *Bilious.*

Aggravation: In the morning: After coffee: On alternate days, a later hour each time. During day: Soon after drinking, especially warm drinks: At night: After rising in morning: 4 A. M.: In old people: In premature old age, with syphilitic-mercurial dyscrasia: Weakly constitutions: After trivial errors of diet.

Before Stool: Viscid, tasteless saliva in the mouth: Burning, pinching pain in the stomach and about the navel: Sensation of distension from flatulence: Griping, severe pain the lower part of abdomen.

During Stool: Protrusion of hæmorrhoids: Prolapsus ani: Pain about the navel: Tenesmus.

After Stool: Abdominal pain; Tenesmus.

Accompaniments: Viscid saliva in the mouth at night on waking. Diminished appetite. Desire for highly-seasoned and piquant things. Aversion to coffee. Feeling of emptiness about the navel, relieved by tightening the clothes. Bilious vomiting after errors in diet. Sensibility to pressure in right hypochondrium. Sallow skin and emaciation. Great loss of memory, much fear and anxiety.

Fluoric acid deserves careful study in chronic diarrhœa, in broken down persons who have had syphilis and have taken much mercury, and in hard drinkers with bad livers.

62. GAMBOGIA.

Stools: *Thin, yellow, fecal;* Watery; Yellowish or greenish watery, mixed with mucus; Dark yellowish-brown, watery; Bloody, mucous or slimy; Dark green mucous; Undigested; Like curdled milk;

Offensive (dark green mucous stool); Corrosive;

Frequent; Quite copious; Odorless (watery mucous);

Coming out all at once, with a single, somewhat prolonged effort. Diarrhœa alternating with constipation.

Aggravation: Forenoon or during the day: After drinking ale: After taking cold: In children: In hot weather: In old people: Mornings: After eating: At night.

Amelioration: From pressing the abdomen (cutting pains).

Before Stool: *Sudden urging, with hot pinching throughout the abdomen:* Darting stitches in anus: Sensation of fulness in the abdomen: Excessive cutting around navel: Constant urging, with colicky pains: Severe pains causing him to draw up limbs and cry out.

During Stool: *Strong urging, causing the stool to pass quickly:* Much flatus: Burning and heat in the anus: Tenesmus: Prolapsus ani: Cutting pain about the navel: Cold sweat on the limbs.

After Stool: **Feeling of great relief in the abdomen, as though an irritating substance were removed from the intestines: Burning in the anus:** Anus sore and excoriated: Sometimes severe pains in lower bowels.

Accompaniments: Despondency. Sadness. Bitter taste in the mouth. Burning of the tongue. Diminished appetite. There seems to be a good appetite, but a little food satisfies it. **Voluptuous itching of the canthi and eyelids; child rubs them often.**

Aphthæ; deep ulcers in the mouth, inner side of the lips and cheeks. Nausea and vomiting, after taking drink or food (with the watery and sometimes the mucous stools).

Rumbling in the abdomen. Gurgling, as of a fluid running from a bottle. Pain and sensitiveness to pressure in the ileo-cœcal region.

Urine smells like onions, scenting the room.

Feeling of soreness all over the body.

Much lassitude and debility. Emaciation.

Gambogia is one of the most important remedies in the treatment of diarrhœa, both acute and chronic, and has also a place in the therapeutics of infantile diarrhœa and of dysentery. It closely resembles **Aloe**. It may be distinguished, however, by the absence of hæmorrhoids, by the rapid expulsion of stool, and by the immediate accompanying symptoms of the stool as italicized above. When well selected, **Gambogia** usually gives a prompt and permanent cure, without subsequent aid from other remedies.

63. GELSEMIUM.

Stools: Yellow fecal; *Cream-colored fecal;* Bilious; Tea green or olive green; Involuntary.

Aggravation: **From sudden depressing emotions, fright, grief, bad news,** *excitement: During dentition:* In the evening (general condition).

Before Stool: Colic: Passage of flatus.

During Stool: Difficult passage of stool, as though the sphincter ani were spasmodically closed.

Accompaniments: Child frantic at times, especially when the gums are examined. Seizes things when carried, as if afraid of falling. Starts up screaming. *Desire to be quiet or to be let alone.* Feeling of intoxication. Gums swollen and tender. Tongue coated yellowish-white, with fetid breath. *Little or no thirst.* Pain in the bowels after beginning to walk, relieved by continued walking. Chilliness in the back. Drowsiness. *Slight fever, with full, round, soft, flowing pulse.*

Many persons are seized with diarrhœa whenever subjected to sudden depressing emotions, particularly fear and anxiety. The anticipation of any unusual ordeal—as appearing in public, undergoing an examination, submitting to a surgical operation—is sufficient to excite it. **Gels.** removes it, together with the trepidation which caused it. It is a short-acting remedy, and, although relieving the attacks, will seldom cure the disposition to them; some carefully chosen antipsoric must do that.

64. GRAPHITES.

Stools: *Brown fluid, mixed with undigested substances, and of an intolerable fetor; Pasty, like mud, adhering to the vessel; Watery.*

Reddish or white mucous; Knotty, lumps united by stringy mucus.

Sour-smelling; Corrosive.

Aggravation: At night: After taking cold: After the menses: Night and morning: From drinking.

Before Stool: Colic.

During Stool: Burning in the rectum: Tenesmus.

After Stool: Smarting soreness in the anus

Tender hæmorrhoids: Great but transient prostration.

Accompaniments: Child impertinent, laughs at reprimands. Bitter taste in the mouth. Taste as of rotten eggs in the morning. Sour taste after a meal. Tongue coated. Aversion to salt things, *meat* and fish. Sweet things cause nausea and disgust. Putrid eructations. Desire for drink to cool one's self internally, without thirst. Fulness and hardness of the abdomen. *Distended abdomen, even after eating but little*, with rush of blood to the head. Urine fetid, sour or turbid, with reddish sediment. Offensive sweat.

Lassitude of the whole body. Inclination to stretch, without being able to satisfy it sufficiently. Great itching, as though fecal matter would pass through the skin. Enlarged glands. Emaciation. Chlorosis.

Graph. occupies a subordinate position in the treatment of diarrhœa, but the emphasized symptoms describe a condition sometimes met with, and often chronic, where it proves curative. It is especially adapted to fat, flabby persons, who suffer from constant chilliness, and are subject to eczematous and herpetic eruptions, which crack and ooze a glutinous fluid. These are apt to occur behind the ears or in the bends of the joints, and are associated with marked absence of perspiration.

65. GRATIOLA OFFICINALIS.

Stools: *Watery; Yellow, green, frothy, watery;* Brown fetid mucous.

Frequent; *Gushing out with force;* Involuntary; Painless; Green fluid gradually changing to colorless.

Aggravation: In the open air: After drinking too freely of water not very cold.

Amelioration: After eating, and by eructations (nausea): By passing flatus (pains).

Before Stool: Nausea: Rumbling in the abdomen: Cutting round the umbilicus.

During Stool: Nausea: Burning pain in rectum: Soreness in anus: Tenesmus.

After Stool: Pressure in the abdomen when walking, disappearing when sitting: Coldness: Shuddering when entering a room: Burning pains in rectum: Burning in anus: Wrenching pains in coccyx: Creeping chills.

Accompaniments: Accumulation of clear water in the mouth, causing frequent spitting. Appetite for nothing but bread. Aversion to smoking. Violent thirst. Nausea, and inclination to vomit. Vomiting of bitter water or a yellowish substance. Violent vomiting, often accompanied by pains in the head, vomiting first of greenish water, later colorless. Cold feeling of the stomach, as if full of water. Much flatulence.

Cold feeling in the abdomen. Severe cramps in abdomen, extending over the whole body.

There is reason to believe that **Gratiola** will prove particularly serviceable in cases of cholera morbus resulting from drinking excessive quantities of water of moderate coolness; the quantity, and not the coldness, being the cause.

66. HELLEBORUS NIGER.

Stools: *White, jelly-like, mucous; Pure, tenacious, white mucous;* Colorless mucous; White gelatinous, like frog's spawn; Watery;

Frequent: Involuntary.

Aggravation: In children: *During dentition:* During acute hydrocephalus: From 4 to 8 P. M.: During pregnancy.

Before Stool: Nausea: Colic.

During Stool: Urging: Tenesmus: Nausea.

After Stool: *Burning, smarting at the anus:* Relief of colic.

Accompaniments: Taciturnity. Rolling of the head. Head hot. Eyes partly open. Eyeballs rolled upward. Pupils dilated and insensible to light. Squinting. Sudden shrieks. Face pale, œdematous, hippocratic; forehead wrinkled. Ptyalism, with soreness of the corners of the mouth. Great thirst. Aphthæ. Much gagging. Vomiting of green or blackish substances.

Urine scanty and dark, with floating black specks, or containing a deposit looking like coffee grounds. Cramps in extremities. Voice weak.

Skin cold and clammy. Pulse often intermittent. Automatic motion of one side of the body.

Hell. n. brings help sometimes, when, without it help would be hard to find, or be sought in vain. The stool is chiefly characteristic, and is such as sometimes occurs in protracted and dangerous cases of infantile diarrhœa.

67. HEPAR SULPHUR.

Stools: *Light yellow fecal; Thin or papescent; Green, watery;* Black; *Undigested; Whitish, sour smelling;* Bloody mucous; *Green, slimy, fetid; Smelling like rotten cheese;*

Painless; Expulsion difficult.

Aggravation: During the day: After eating: after drinking cold water: After abuse of mercury or cinchona: In dyspeptics.

Amelioration: *After eating* (symptoms of the stomach).

Accompaniments: Depressed or irritable mood. Disinclination for mental or bodily exertion. Sourish, metallic taste. Bitter taste. Generally good appetite. Desire for acids; wine; tea. *Craving for condiments.* Much thirst. Hot, *sour regurgitation of food.* Sour vomiting. Vomiting of green, acrid water. Frequent momentary attacks of nausea. Morning nausea and vomiting. Pressure and pain in the stomach, relieved by eating; by eructation; by passing flatus. *Empty, sinking feeling at the stomach. Strong and comfortable feeling after a meal. Frequent desire* *to loosen the clothing about the stomach*, particularly a few hours after a meal. Acrid feeling in the stomach during digestion. Bruised sore feeling of the body, worse from any motion. *The child smells sour.* Swollen glands.

Desire to be covered even in a warm room.

Over-sensitiveness to pain.

Hepar sul. occupies a leading position in the therapeutics of chronic diarrhœa. The cases calling for it are among the most common. They come often from allopathic treatment, having abuse of mercury or cinchona, and often suppression of scabies in their history. So many of the characteristic symptoms are referred to the stomach, that the cases might be classed under dyspepsia. It most resembles **Lycop.** The time of aggravation is the most constant distinction. A comfortable feeling after eating is very characteristic.

68. HIPPOMANE MANCINELLA.

Stools: Dark or black fecal, afterward watery; Fetid.

Aggravation: At night: At midnight: In the morning: After drinking water (colic).

Before Stool: Sudden urging: Colic.

During Stool: Colic: Much discharge of flatus: burning in the stomach and anus: Tenesmus.

After Stool: Pulsation in the anus.

Accompaniments: Violent headache. Dryness of the mouth. Burning in the mouth, not relieved by cold water. Mouth and tongue studded with small vesicles, preventing the taking of solid nourishment. Bleeding of the mouth. Tongue coated white, with small red spots not coated. Bloody taste. Bitter taste, worse after sleeping. Increased saliva, fetid, yellowish, burning. Thirst for water. Aversion to wine spirits, meat and bread. Violent vomiting of ingesta; bitter; watery; green; *of a bitter watery substance, on which float pieces like white, hardened fat.*

Tympanitis. Drowsiness.

Though published over thirty-four years ago, this remedy remains a stranger to most of us. The symptoms are not at all equivocal, and it may well be placed among our reserve forces.

69. HYDROPHOBIN.

Stools: Bloody mucous; Bloody; Watery; Profuse.

Aggravation: *On seeing water, or hearing it run:* At night; In morning.

Amelioration: By sipping tea.

During Stool: Tenesmus.

After Stool: Tenesmus; Pain in the rectum and small of back; Nausea.

Accompaniments: Ill humor. Irritability. Inclination to be rude and abusive, to bite and strike. Aversion to drinking water, but can take small quantities of chocolate. Large quantities of tough saliva in the mouth, with constant spitting.

Hydroph. adds an interesting and well-confirmed symptom to our repertory, in the aggravation, which, with the other symptoms, makes it applicable in dysentery. Those who have scruples about using a remedy of this character are at liberty to cure cases having this distinctive condition with some other remedy if they can.

It has been found useful in chronic cramp diarrhœa.

70. HYOSCYAMUS.

Stools: *Yellow watery;* Watery; Mucous;
Frequent; *Involuntary; In bed without consciousness of it; Painless; Nearly odorless.*

Aggravation: *During typhoid fever:* During pregnancy: In child-bed: When urinating: At night.

Accompaniments: Muttering delirium. Delirium about usual employments; wants to get up and attend to business or go home. Makes abrupt, short answers to imaginary questions. Raises head from pillow and gazes about. *Things seem too large.* Frequent looking at the hands, because they seem too large. Unconsciousness, with no wants except thirst. Fear of being poisoned or sold. When spoken to replies properly, but delirium and unconsciousness immediately return. *Desire to uncover or undress, and remain naked.* Bright, staring eyes. Dilated pupils. Face flushed. Teeth encrusted with brown mucus.

Clean, parched, dry tongue. Much thirst. Hiccough, with spasms and rumbling in the abdomen and foam at the mouth.

Urine scanty or retained, or passed involuntarily in bed, **leaving streaks of red sand on the sheets.**

Sleeplessness from nervous irritation.

Subsultus tendinum. *Picking at the bed-clothes.* Convulsions. Spasms. Attack comes on suddenly without apparent cause.

The symptoms of the stools of **Hyos.** are sufficiently unlike those of any other remedy to make the choice easy, but the accompanying symptoms make it certain.

71. IGNATIA.

Stools: Yellowish-white, slimy; Thin; Pasty; Mucous; Bloody mucous; Acrid; Sometimes painless; Involuntary (when passing flatus); Alternate diarrhœa and constipation.

Aggravation: During dentition: *In nervous, hysterical persons:* After fright: After eating: At night: When standing (constriction of the anus): After coffee and tobacco and from emotions (general condition).

Before Stool: Rumbling: Urging, felt mostly in the middle and upper abdomen.

During Stool: Prolapsus recti: Smarting in the anus: Passing much flatus.

After Stool: Prolapsus recti: *Tenesmus:* Constriction of the anus, worse when standing: Great nervous erethism.

Accompaniments: *Suppressed grief, with over-sensitiveness. Alternate laughing and crying.* Great timidity. Frequent sighing. Child has much sobbing, sighing and crying. Sobbing and sighing continue long after the crying has ceased. Face pale, clay-colored, sunken, with blue rings around the eyes; or alternately red and pale; or redness and heat of one cheek and ear. Eructations of bitter fluid or food into the mouth. Hiccough after eating and drinking and after emotions. Nausea, usually without vomiting. Hunger and nausea at the same time. Hunger in the evening prevents sleep. *Empty retching, relieved by eating.* Aversion to tobacco, warm food, meat and spirituous liquors. *Empty, sinking feeling at the stomach, with qualmishness, flat taste and desire to draw a long breath. Urine frequent, watery, profuse.* Child awakens from sleep with piercing cries and trembles all over. Frequent flushes of heat, with perspiration. Convulsive jerks of single parts.

Spasms: from difficult dentition; preceded by hasty drinking; return at the same hour daily; trembling all over; cries and involuntary laughter.

Ignatia is not often indicated in acute diseases of the bowels, but is valuable in certain forms of diarrhœa and dysentery, characterized by great nervous erethism and tenesmus occurring only after stool. The italicized accompaniments are very characteristic, especially the desire to take a deep breath to relieve the sinking at the stomach.

72. IODINE.

Stools: *Watery, foamy, whitish mucous;* **Whey-like;** *Fatty;*

Bloody, mucous; Thick, mucous; Fecal; *Purulent;* Copious; Fetid; Alternation of constipation and diarrhœa.

Aggravation: *In the morning:* After milk: After eating (abdominal symptoms): *In a warm room* (general condition): In old people.

Amelioration: *After eating* (pain in stomach).

Before Stool: Severe pain as though being stepped on, in whole abdomen, relieved in no position.

During Stool: Cutting pain in the bowels.

After Stool: Burning at the anus.

Accompaniments: *Restlessness. Inclination to constantly change position, so that one can neither sit nor sleep.* Children very irritable, will not allow anyone to approach them. Fear of being touched. Pressive pains in the vertex. Pale, yellowish complexion. Aphthæ in the mouth, with ptyalism. Thickly coated or dry tongue. Putrid smell from the mouth. Sour taste in the mouth. Much thirst. *Eating too often and too much, digestion being rapid, and yet the emaciation goes on.* Pains in the stomach, gnawing or corroding, better after eating. Violent and continued vomiting, renewed by eating. Left hypochondrium hard and painful on pressure (enlarged spleen). Cutting in the abdomen. Incarceration of flatus in left abdomen. Pressing and bearing down toward the pelvis. Enlargement of the mesenteric glands. Urine ammoniacal. *Palpitation of the heart, worse from the least exertion.* Sleeplessness. *Emaciation.* Prostration and debility.

Iodine is suitable mostly to a chronic diarrhœa of an exhausting character and in persons with dark eyes and hair. The restlessness is a constant desire for change of place, without anguish and tossing, as in **Ars.**

73. IPECACUANHA.

Stools: *Green mucous,* **as green as grass;** Lumpy, greenish, watery; Lemon-colored; White, mucous; *Bloody;* Bloody, mucous; *Fermented;* Bilious; *Dark, almost black, looking like frothy molasses;*

Putrid; Frequent.

Aggravation: At night: In the evening: During dentition: In children: After a cold: From motion (colic): In the autumn: After unripe fruit or vegetables: After eating sour substances: From anger, mortification or vexation, with indignation: In fat, pale children.

Amelioration: From rest (colic).

Before Stool: *Colic: Nausea:* Vomiting.

During Stool: Colic: *Nausea:* Vomiting: Coldness: Paleness: Violent tenesmus (dysenteric stools).

After Stool: Lassitude: Tenesmus (dysenteric stools): Twitching of face.

Accompaniments: Irritability. Impatience. Open fontanelles. *Pale face*, with blue margins about the eyes, and constant look of nausea. Pupils dilated. Epistaxis, with pale face. *Cold sweat on the forehead. Tongue clean.* Increased secretion of saliva. Loathing of food. No thirst. Desire for dainties and sweet things. **Nausea**, proceeding from the stomach, with empty eructations and a flow of saliva, with pale face and suppressed breathing.

Vomiting: immediately after eating; after drinking; of ingesta; of yellow mucus; of bile; of large lumps of fetid mucus; *of green, jelly-like mucus; of grass-green mucus;* of large quantities of mucus. Excessive, indescribable sick feeling in the region of the stomach. *Flatulent colic.* Griping, pinching about the umbilicus, as though the intestines were grasped with hands. Skin cool. Oppressed breathing. Suffocative catarrh of the chest. Spasms. Sleep with eyes half open. Drowsiness, with starting and jerking of the muscles during sleep.

The continuous nausea is the most constant distinctive symptom of **Ipec**. The addition of the characteristic vomiting and the violent colic is more rare, and renders the choice more nearly certain. This remedy is seldom suited to cases of long continuance, and is often unable to complete the cure alone. In cholera infantum it may need to be followed by **Arsenicum**.

74. IRIS VERSICOLOR.

Stools: Brown; *Watery;* Watery, mixed with mucus;

Bloody, mucous; Thin, yellow, fecal; Black; Mushy; Papescent;

Greenish; Undigested; Involuntary;

Frequent; Profuse; Corrosive; Fetid or coppery-smelling.

Aggravation: At night: After supper: *At 2 or 3 A.M.:* In hot weather: In children (in Spring and Autumn).

Amelioration: By bending double (colic) and passing flatus.

Before Stool: Rumbling in the abdomen: Cutting in the lower part of the abdomen.

During Stool: Cutting: Severe cramp-like pains: *Tenesmus:* **Burning at the anus**: *Fetid*, coppery-smelling flatus.

After Stool: Pricking as of points in the anus: **Burning of the anus, as though on fire**: *Prolapse of the rectum.*

Accompaniments: Despondency. Severe headache. Sunken eyes. Flat taste. Bitter or putrid taste. Increase of saliva, which is ropy. **Burning from the mouth to the anus**. White tongue. Loss of appetite. Empty eructations. *Nausea. Vomiting, with burning in mouth, fauces and œsophagus.* Violent vomiting of ingesta; of bile; **of an extremely sour fluid, which excoriates the throat.** Violent efforts to vomit, resulting in enormous forcible eructations. Violent pain with every fit of vomiting. Great burning distress in stomach. Pain in umbilical region, with loud rumbling in the bowels. Tympanitis. Burning in the urethra after micturition. Cramps. Fever, with hot sweat. *Much exhaustion and debility from the first.* Limbs and body cold.

The characteristic symptoms of **Iris v.** are not among those of most frequent occurrence, but when met with are not difficult to recognize. It will be found applicable mostly to cholera morbus, occurring in the hottest of the season. It is said to have been used successfully in cholera, with icy-cold tongue and general coldness of the surface.

75. JABORANDI.

Stools: Thin, yellow, watery, undigested; *Gushing; Painless.*

Aggravation: During the day (mostly between 6 A.M. and noon): At noon (headache).

Amelioration: By eating (distress in the stomach).

Accompaniments: Headache. *Face flushed.* **Profuse salivation.** *Intense thirst.* Great nausea and retching, often attended with hiccough and sometimes terminating in vomiting. Eructations. Distress in the stomach, relieved by eating. Empty, gone feeling in the abdomen. *Urine dark, scanty* or profuse. Rapid pulse, with visible throbbing of the arteries. **Profuse sweat.**

The symptoms of **Jaborandi** are so peculiar and striking that this remedy may well be placed among our reserve forces for future study and verification.

76. JALAPA.

Stools: *Watery; Sour-smelling; Bloody.*

Aggravation: In infants: At night.

Before and During Stool: *Cutting colic.*

Accompaniments: *Great restlessness and anxiety.*

Nausea and vomiting.

Severe griping, cutting pains in the bowels, worse at night.

Child is quiet all day, but screams and tosses about all night. General coldness, with blueness of the face.

Jalapa is very valuable for severe nightly colic of infants, with or without diarrhœa.

77. JATROPHA CURCAS.

Stools: *Watery;*
Profuse gushing out like a torrent.

Accompaniments: Apathy. *Indifference to pain;* or anxiety and anguish. Pale face, blue margins about the eyes. Dryness and burning of the mouth, tongue and throat, or increase of thin saliva. Violent, *unquenchable thirst*. Eructations. Vomiting of large masses of dark green bile and mucus, **of large quantities of watery, albuminous substances**. Burning in the stomach. Spasmodically contracting pains in the stomach. Abdomen swollen and tender to the touch. Rumbling *and noise as of a bottle of water being emptied* in the abdomen, not ceasing after stool. *Violent cramps in the legs and feet. Coldness of the body. General cold, clammy perspiration.*

Those who have used **Jatropha** in the treatment of cholera have confirmed the above symptoms, and they are such as give it a prominent place in the treatment of the first stage of that disease, before the period of collapse. The albuminous vomiting is very characteristic. This and the other symptoms are also sometimes met with in cholera morbus.

In some respects it resembles **Ipec.**, but may be distinguished from the latter remedy by the burning thirst and violent cramps.

78. KALI BICHROMICUM.

Stools: Blackish, watery; Yellowish, watery; Clay-colored, watery and lumpy; *Brownish, frothy, watery; Bloody; Jelly-like;*

Frequent; Gushing out (watery stools); Involuntary and often painless and odorless.

Aggravation: *In the morning: Periodically, every year:* In the early part of the summer:

After rheumatism: *From lager beer: In fat, light-haired persons.*

Before Stool: *Urgent pressure to stool* (waking one in the morning).

During Stool: *Painful urging: Tenesmus: Gnawing pain about the umbilicus.*

After Stool: *Tenesmus:* Burning in the abdomen, with nausea and violent straining to vomit.

Accompaniments: Ill humor. Sadness. Pale, yellowish complexion. Small scabs on the septum of the nose. Dryness of the mouth and lips, relieved only a short time by taking water. Increase of saliva, which is frothy, viscid, and tastes bitter or salty. *Tongue coated thick, brown, like thick, yellow felt at the root, papillæ elevated. Large insular patches on the tongue.* **Tongue dry, red, smooth and cracked.** Much thirst. Desire for ale or acid drinks. Nausea, with feeling of heat in the whole body and dizziness. Vomiting of sour, undigested food; of bitter bile; of mucus; of pinkish, *stringy*, glairy fluid; of blood; accompanied by cold perspiration on the hands. Tympanitis. Gnawing pain about the umbilicus. Stitches in the right side of the chest and in the left sciatic nerve.

Much debility and desire to lie down.

Kali bichr. proves of great service in a variety of cases, but chiefly in dysentery, with the characteristic tongue and gelatinous stools. Sometimes, however, with those stools the tongue has nothing peculiar. The morning aggravation will then decide the choice. After **Canth.** has removed stools like scrapings, jelly-like stools will sometimes appear. **Kali bichr.** will then complete the cure. It is also valuable in chronic morning diarrhœa and chronic clay-colored diarrhœa.

79. KALI BROMICUM.

Stools. Watery (like rice-water); Frequent; Green; Bloody; Muco-purulent;

Painless.

During Stool: Sensation as if the bowels were falling out: Dribbling of urine.

Accompaniments: Anxiety and restlessness. Rolling of head. Hot head. Pale face.

Eyes sunken and congested. Pupils dilated. Convulsive motion of eyes and limbs. Eyeballs moving in every direction without taking any notice.

Mouth dry. Intense thirst. Thrush in mouth.

Internal coldness of the abdomen.

Colicky pains in the abdomen.

Sensation as if the bowels were falling out. Violent abdominal spasms, during which abdomen gets very hard.

Urine scanty, dribbling a few drops at the beginning of every stool.

Burning in the chest.

Pulse rapid and weak, imperceptible.

Shaking of the body as if from palsy. **Feet** and hands blue and cold.

Great chilliness, even in a hot room.

Emaciation. Night terror during dentition. Starts, jactitations, spasms.

Kali brom. deserves further clinical observation. It has been used successfully in cholera infantum, with great prostration, coldness of the surface and symptoms of hydrocephaloid.

80. KALI CARBONICUM.

Stools: *Light gray, fecal;* Yellowish or brown, fecal; Alternating with constipation; Corrosive; Sometimes painless;

Profuse; Involuntary (when passing flatus).

Aggravation: At night: At 3 or 4 A. M.: During the day: In the evening: Day and night: After milk.

Before Stool: Sudden and violent urging: Colic: Pinching deep in the abdomen: *Rumbling*.

During Stool: Colic: Smarting at the anus: Nausea.

After Stool: *Burning at the anus:* Pinching pains.

Accompaniments: Irritable. Easily startled. Aversion to noise. *Hair dry, rapidly falling off, with much dandruff*. Face yellow, bloated. **Swelling over the upper eyelids in the morning, like a little bag.** One cheek hot, the other cold. *Bitter taste*. Desire for acids or sugar. Aversion to rye bread or brown bread. Sour eructations. Sour vomiting. Stitches in region of liver, with tension across the abdomen. Icterus. Much flatulence. Abdomen hard, bloated and sensitive about the umbilicus, with pain in the back. Stitching pains, extending from the back into the gluteal muscles. Sharp, shooting, stitching pains all over the abdomen. Drowsiness in the daytime and early in the evening. Much weariness. Debility and desire to lie down. Weak pulse.

Kali c. is only useful in chronic cases, with the peculiar cachexia revealed by the puffiness under the eyebrow.

81. KALI NITRICUM.

Stools: Watery; Thin, fecal; Bloody.

Aggravation: In the morning: During the day: *After eating veal*.

Amelioration: By emission of flatus (colic and urging).

Before Stool: Violent colic: Urging.

During Stool: Cutting colic in whole intestinal canal: Tenesmus.

After Stool: Cutting colic: Tenesmus: Burning and stinging in the anus.

Accompaniments: Headache. Fetid odor from the mouth. Tongue coated white. Little appetite, with much thirst. Violent colic, more in the right side of the abdomen.

Debility, felt more when sitting than during gentle motion.

Some persons always have diarrhœa after eating veal. The curability of such cases with **Kali nitr.** needs somewhat more confirmation, but no other remedy has had this symptom so well confirmed as yet.

82. KREOSOTUM.

Stools: *Greenish or chopped; Greenish, watery; Dark brown, watery;* Grayish; White; Papescent; Undigested; *Fetid; Cadaverous-smelling;* Excoriating.

Aggravation: In nursing infants: During dentition: From 6 P. M. until 6 A. M. (general condition): In tall, delicate, blonde children: In old women.

Accompaniments: Great irritability. Blueness around the nose, temples and mouth. *Very painful dentition. Gums hot, swollen, tender, and look as if infiltrated with a dark, watery fluid.* **Teeth show dark specks and begin to decay as soon as they appear.** Tongue coated white. *Craving for smoked meats.* Intense thirst, with greedy drinking. *Continuous vomiting and straining to vomit.* Vomiting of food for several hours after it has been eaten. *Vomiting in the evening of all food eaten during the day.* Belching and hiccoughing when carried. Griping about the navel. Abdomen distended. Child resists the tightening of anything about the abdomen which increases the restlessness and pain. Dreams that he is urinating, and awakes to find the dream a reality. Hands and feet cold. Very restless, tossing about all night; *will only sleep when caressed and fondled;* moaning and dozing with half-open eyes. Quick, scarcely perceptible pulse. Exhaustion and rapid emaciation.

Although not one of the most frequently indicated remedies, **Kreos.** occupies an important place in our therapia. The symptoms of the teeth and gums are especially characteristic. It is followed well by **Sulphur.** After **Carbo veg.** it disagrees.

83. LACHESIS.

Stools: Watery; Light yellow, fecal; Purulent; Thin, pasty; *Chocolate-colored; Consisting of decomposed blood* **looking like charred straw;** *Bloody water;* Bloody and slimy;

Very offensive; Cadaverous-smelling; Undigested; Frequent; Corrosive;

Involuntary; Alternating with constipation.

Aggravation: After eating or drinking: *In the spring;* In warm weather: In the evening or night: After acids: After fruit: During typhoid fever: **After sleep:** Before or after menses: In drunkards: During climaxis.

Amelioration: By bending forward (colic).

Before Stool: Rumbling: Urging.

During Stool: Burning at the anus: Tenesmus.

After Stool: Burning at the anus: Tenesmus: Protrusion of large hæmorrhoidal tumors, with constriction of the anus and continued desire for stool: Throbbing as with little hammers in anus.

Accompaniments: Loquacity. *Anterior half of the tongue red, smooth and shining; cracked at the tip;* or tongue black and bloody. Vesicles on the tip of the tongue.

In putting out the tongue it catches on the teeth or under-lip. Much thirst. Desire for wine; for oysters. *Desire to loosen the clothing about the waist.* Spasmodic colic, relieved by bending forward. Much flatulence. Loud eructations which relieve the stomach. Distension of the abdomen. Cramp-like pains in the abdomen, which feels hot. *Tenderness in the left iliac region, with intolerance of the slightest pressure.* Frothy urine. *Languor. Debility.* Exhaustion as from warm weather. Shivering without coldness. *Much distress after sleep.*

Lach. is not often required in the treatment of diarrhœa. In chronic cases, or when occurring in the progress of other acute diseases, it may become indicated by the concomitant symptoms.

84. LAUROCERASUS.

Stools: *Green, liquid, mucous;* Fecal; *Green watery;* Yellowish, mushy, undigested;

Involuntary.

Aggravation: In the afternoon: After cold food: After eating or drinking (pains).

Before Stool: Cutting in the abdomen.

During Stool: Tenesmus: Loud emission of flatus.

After Stool: Burning at the anus.

Accompaniments: Sunken countenance. Livid, grayish-yellow complexion. Eyes staring, or lightly closed; *pupils dilated* (sometimes contracted and immovable). White and dry tongue. Violent thirst. Entire loss of appetite. Sensation of constriction in the throat when swallowing. **Drink rolls audibly through the œsophagus and intestines.** Severe pain in the bowels. Stitching pain in the liver. Distension of the region of the liver, which is very tender to the touch. Indurated liver.

Suppression or retention of urine.

Slow, feeble, moaning or rattling breathing.

Irregular action of the heart, with suffocative attacks and great anguish in the cardiac region.

Pulse slow, irregular or imperceptible.

Skin cold, livid.

In Cholera: *Absence of vomiting and stools: Asphyxia: Coldness of the body:* Pulselessness: Fainting: Tetanic spasms: Staring, fixed look: Dilated pupils: Respiration slow, deep, gasping, difficult and spasmodic, at long intervals.

The symptoms of **Lauroc.** remind us at once of a most severe and fatal form of cholera infantum. The rattling of drink as it rolls down the œsophagus is the most characteristic symptom, and one of evil omen. In these cases, the other symptoms corresponding, this remedy will save many otherwise fatal cases. The same remark applies also to cholera and cholera morbus.

85. LEPTANDRA.

Stools: *Black, fecal fluid, running from the bowels in a stream; Black, papescent, tar-like; Yellowish green;* Watery; Watery mucous; Watery, with large quantities of mucus; Greenish, muddy, watery, spouting out like water; Mucous, bilious and bloody; Consisting of pure blood; *Profuse; Fetid;* Excoriating; Undigested.

Aggravation: In the morning after rising and moving about: In the afternoon and evening: From meat or vegetables.

Before Stool: Great urging, with inability to retain the stool: Severe colic: Loud rumbling and gurgling in the abdomen as of water.

After Stool: *Sharp, cutting pains and distress in the umbilical region:* Weak feeling in the abdomen and rectum: Faintness: Hunger.

Accompaniments: Face sallow. Tongue coated yellow along the centre. Nausea, with faintness. Vomiting. *Severe and constant distress between the umbilicus and epigastrium*, with sharp, cutting pains. Aching, burning sensation in the region of the liver, aggravated by drinking cold water. Brown urine.

Much distress.

Clinically, little is known of **Lept.**; but the symptoms derived from provings are peculiar and distinctive, though not such as are often met with in practice. The symptom of the region of the liver is found on the opposite side, under **Natr.**

carb. The griping colic after stool without tenesmus will distinguish **Lept.** from **Merc. sol.**

86. LILIUM TIGRINUM.

Stools: Dark brown, semi-liquid fecal; Copious, bilious; Bloody, mucous;

Very offensive.

Aggravation: In the morning and forenoon:

In the evening until midnight (general condition):

When standing (bearing down).

Before Stool: Peremptory urging: Constant dragging, bearing down sensation, with pressure in the rectum producing continual desire for stool.

During Stool: Tenesmus of the bladder and rectum.

After Stool: Acrid smarting and burning in the rectum and anus: Severe tenesmus: Exhaustion.

Accompaniments: *Constant hurried feeling as if imperative duties demanded attention, with inability to perform them.* Depression of spirits. Apprehension of some approaching disease. Excitement and defiance under restraint. Loss of appetite. Aversion to coffee and bread. Abdomen feels bloated and is tender. Trembling sensation in the abdomen. Frequent desire to urinate, with smarting in the urethra during micturition; urine high-colored and scanty. *Pressure downward through the pelvis, as if everything would push out, with desire to press upward on the peri-*

neum and vulva. Dragging down sensation extending to the hypogastrium, thorax and shoulders, with aching and dragging in the back. Burning in the pelvis. Stitching pains from ilium to ilium or from pubis to sacrum. Sharp burning pains and stitches in the ovaries, which are swollen and tender, especially during the menses. Sexual excitement. Hands and feet cold and clammy when excited.

The value of **Lilium tig.** in morning diarrhœa, associated with, or dependent upon, prolapsus uteri and ovarian irritation, has been confirmed by abundant clinical observation.

87. LITHIUM CARBONICUM.

Stools: Light, yellow, fecal;
Stinking.
Aggravation: *After fruit: After chocolate: At night:* In the morning.
Accompaniments: Appetite quickly satisfied. *Gnawing pains in the stomach, relieved by eating.*
Emission of much offensive flatus waking one from sleep. Pain in the bladder before and after urination. Strong urging to urinate.

88. LYCOPODIUM.

Stools: Thin, brown or pale fecal, mixed with hard lumps; *Thin yellow or reddish yellow fluid;* Shaggy, reddish mucous; Undigested; Purulent; Bloody; Green; Offensive (green);
Painless: Painful (dysenteric stools).

Aggravation: *At 4 P. M. and until 8 P. M. (flatulence, pains and stools):* At 1 A. M., or soon after midnight, or 2 to 3 A. M. (stools): During pregnancy: After milk: After oysters (?): *After a meal (stomach and abdomen): In the morning (stools):* After cold food: After suppressed eruptions (especially scabies).

Amelioration: (Of the stomach symptoms): By eructations: *By loosening the clothing about the stomach:* By stroking the epigastrium with the hand: By application of cold substances to the epigastrium: *After eating*.

Before Stool: Chilliness in the rectum: Colic.

During Stool: Biting at the anus: Burning at the anus: Chilliness: Colic: Distressing pressure in the rectum: Tenesmus.

After Stool: Sense of insufficient evacuation (dysenteric stools).

Accompaniments: Child sad and listless, or nervous, irritable and unmanageable. Earthy color of the face. Flushed face. Blue rings around the eyes. Eyes wide open, fixed, insensible to light. Child does not wink. Bad or putrid smell from the mouth in the morning. Bitter taste. Sour taste in the mouth, and of food. Little or no thirst. Canine hunger. Desire for sweet things. Aversion to bread; to warm, boiled food; to meat; to coffee; to smoking. If the canine hunger be not satisfied, severe headache results, which is relieved after eating. **A little food seems to fill the stomach full, and causes**

fulness and distension of the abdomen. *Eructations. Pain, tenderness and swelling of the region of the stomach, relieved by loosening the clothing.* Sinking at the stomach.

Nausea in the morning. *Flatulent distension of the abdomen.* Constant sense of fermentation in the abdomen. Abdominal walls so sensitive that laughing is painful.

Incarcerated flatulence. Loud rumbling of flatus in the abdomen, especially in the left hypochondrium. Child cries before urinating. *Urine deposits red sand on the diaper.* Suppression of urine.

Fatigue in the thighs, which no position relieves: desire to stretch them apart and then press them together again. *Fatigue and weakness is felt more during rest than during motion. Heat between the scapulæ.* Child sleeps with half-open eyes and throws its head from side to side, with moaning.

Sleep disturbed by frequent waking; child springs up terrified and screaming, *and is angry and cross, striking, kicking and scratching every one who approaches.* Desire to go into the open air.

Weakness. *Nervous debility.*

Chlorosis. Emaciation.

Feet cold. One foot hot, the other cold.

Spasms, with screaming, foaming at the mouth; unconsciousness, throwing the arms about.

Lycop. is one of the noblest monuments to the

genius of Hahnemann, as well as one of the most convincing proofs of the homœopathic doctrines. This innocent substance is developed by potentizing into one of our most valuable remedies for chronic diarrhœa, as met with in weak, chlorotic, dyspeptic and debilitated persons. The characteristic symptoms are marked, and need no comment. The symptoms of the stool are subordinate. The "chilliness in the rectum," before stool, is a singular but genuine symptom, which further observation may prove to be characteristic. It should be thought of in cholera infantum, with brain symptoms.

Before **Lyc.** is frequently needed some other, not antipsoric remedy (often **Nux. vom**).

89. MAGNESIA CARBONICA.

Stools: *Green, watery, frothy,* **with green scum like that of a frog-pond;** *White lumps, like masses of tallow, floating in the green, watery stool; Bloody mucous;* Green mucous; Greenish-yellow, slimy, mucous; Brown, fluid;

Profuse; *Sour-smelling;* Undigested (containing curdled milk).

Aggravation: In hot weather: During dentition: During the day: After fruit: From artificial foods.

Amelioration: After eating warm soup (colic).

Before Stool: *Cutting and pinching in the abdomen:* General heat: Rumbling: Emission of flatus.

During Stool: Colic: Urging: *Tenesmus*.

After Stool: *Tenesmus:* Burning at the anus.

Accompaniments: Anxiety and general feeling of heat. Bitter taste. Sour taste. Tongue coated white. Aphthæ. Much thirst for cold water, more in the evening and night; also for acid drinks. Desire for fruit. Little appetite. Milk is refused, or if taken causes pain in the stomach. Sour vomiting. Flatulent distension of the abdomen, with rumbling, and cutting and pinching colic. *Sour smell of the whole body*.

Debility.

Much of the ground which should have been occupied by **Magn. carb.** has heretofore been given to **Colc.** and **Merc.** A better acquaintance with the former will prevent this in the future. It is a remedy of the first order in dysentery and infantile diarrhœa. The stools are highly characteristic. The bloody mucus is found mixed with the green, watery stool, sinking to the bottom of the vessel and adhering there; but the watery stool occurs alone.

It follows **Rheum** well, and is often required after that remedy to complete the cure.

90. MERCURIUS CORROSIVUS.

Stools: *Bloody, slimy; Containing shreds of mucous membrane; Offensive;* Yellow, green bilious; Great quantity of pure blood; *Scanty; Frequent*.

Aggravation: Day and night: By motion

(pains and tenesmus): In the fall: After midnight.

Before, during and after Stool: *Constant tenesmus and urging to stool;* Cutting colic.

Accompaniments: *Cold face and hands, with small, feeble pulse.* Astringent, metallic taste. Tongue red and sore. Aphthæ. Ptyalism. Unquenchable thirst. Vomiting of albuminous matter, of tough or stringy mucus, of green, bitter substance. Distension and soreness of pit of stomach not permitting least touch, even of the clothing. Abdomen swollen, hard and sensitive to pressure, especially about the umbilicus.

Tenesmus vesicæ, with intense burning in the urethra, and discharge of mucus and blood, with the urine or after it. Urine scanty, hot, bloody, retained or suppressed.

Stitches in the side. Cramps in the calves.

Limbs feel bruised. Trembling of the limbs. *Faintness, weakness and shuddering.*

In the absence of any provings except poisonings, the finer shades of **Merc. corr.** are not known. One thing is certain, however, that it is too frequently employed in dysentery, to which it is only applicable when occurring in great intensity and accompanied by the characteristic urinary symptoms, as given above. It follows **Acon.** well.

91. MERCURIUS SOLUBILIS.

(*Mercurius vivus.*)

Stools: *Dark green, bilious, frothy;* Like stirred eggs; Brownish; Greenish-brown; *Watery and colorless; Black;* Yellowish; Grayish; *Watery, with greenish scum floating on the surface of the water;* Whitish, watery; Reddish, mucous; *Green, mucous; Bloody mucous; Green, slimy; Bloody; Blood-streaked;* Slimy and fecal; Purulent; *Undigested; Frequent; Scanty; Corrosive; Sour-smelling;* Black, tenacious, like pitch; Hot gushing (yellow fluid).

Aggravation: *From cool evening air:* At night: *In hot weather:* During the day: *During dentition: In cold, damp weather:* After sweats: *While walking.*

Amelioration: By lying down (colic): By standing still (urging).

Before Stool: Sudden urging: *Violent and frequent urging: Nausea:* Pinching and cutting in the abdomen: Anxiety, anguish, trembling and sweat, either warm or cold: *Chilliness:* Chilliness mingled with flashes of heat: Trembling of the whole body.

During Stool: *Violent and frequent urging: Nausea* and vomiting: *Eructations:* Pinching and cutting colic, making one bend double: Burning at the anus: *Chilliness:* Hot sweat on the forehead: *Violent tenesmus: Screaming.*

After Stool: Violent tenesmus and continued

urging: **Never-get-done feeling:** Cutting and pinching colic: Rawness, burning and itching of the anus and adjacent parts: Sensation of constriction in the rectum causing faintness: The pains in the rectum sometimes extend to the back: **Prolapsus recti, the rectum looking dark and bloody:** The warm sweat on the forehead becomes cold: Debility, hiccough, belching.

Accompaniments: Anxious and restless in the evening, with flushed face and hurried speech. Indifference and stupidity. Stammering, owing to trembling of mouth and tongue. Open fontanelles. Large head. Face pale, earthy, yellow. Eyes dull. Gums swollen, bleeding easily. *Tongue swollen, soft and flabby, taking impressions of the teeth on the edges;* coated whitish, yellowish; or dry, hard and black. Aphthæ. *Increase of saliva, or profuse salivation. Bad smell from the mouth. Teeth feel too long and are sensitive.* Taste bitter; putrid. *Desire for butter, for fat food.* Canine hunger. Desire for milk. Aversion to meat, to greasy food.

Violent thirst: for cold drinks; for beer.

Nausea, with vertigo, dimness of vision and flashes of heat. Vomiting, but not for some time after eating. Vomiting of bile; of bitter mucus.

Cutting, griping, stabbing, doubling-up pains in the abdomen, worse at night. Cutting stitch from right to left in the hypogastrium, aggravated by walking. Abdomen cold to the touch.

Region of liver painful and sensitive to contact.

Frequent urination. Tenesmus vesicæ. Urine scanty and turbid, or too profuse or involuntary.

Great debility.

Perspiration on the least exertion. Children restless, with frequent drawing up of the feet and whining.

Thighs and legs cold and clammy, particularly at night. Rheumatic pains in the limbs, worse at night.

Sleeplessness at night, with sleepiness in the daytime. *Restless sleep. Oily, offensive or sour-smelling night-sweat, particularly on the head, cold on the forehead.*

Jaundice. Glands swollen and suppurating.

Few remedies require more careful selection than **Merc.** Its symptoms, though marked and decided, differ more from other remedies in intensity than in quality, and it requires an observing experience to measure this difference. It differs negatively, however, from many other similar remedies, wanting characteristics which they possess. In psoric infants the choice has often to be made between **Calc., Sil.** and **Merc.**, and must be made with care, as a mistake is not easily rectified.

Sil. and **Merc.** do not follow each other well.

92. MEZEREUM.

Stools: Watery; Brown, fecal; *Fermented; Undigested;* Containing small glittering grains; Small; Frequent; *Sour; Offensive.*

Aggravation: In the evening: *After suppression of an eruption of thick crusts covering thick pus.*

Before Stool: *Chill:* Colic: Passing much fetid flatus.

During Stool: Increased urging: Colic: Prolapsus recti: Anus becomes painful and constricted about the fallen rectum.

After Stool: *Chill:* Constriction of the prolapsus: Weakness: Sensitiveness to cold, open air: Painful tenesmus, extending to the perineum and urethra (male).

Accompaniments: Pale, wretched look. Gray, earthy complexion. Increase of saliva. Tongue coated white or yellow. Bitter taste. Desire for ham fat, coffee, wine. Much colic; cutting; pinching, drawing, relieved by rising, stretching and emission of flatus. Exhaustion. Debility.

In cases of chronic diarrhœa, with a psoric anamnesis, **Mez.** will sometimes prove to be the remedy for the whole condition.

It resembles **Merc.** somewhat, and is useful when **Merc.** has been improperly given, and sometimes is needed after **Bellad.**

93. MURIATIC ACID.

Stools: Fecal; *Watery;* Bloody and slimy, separated; Dark brownish-green, gelatinous; Profuse;

Involuntary (without desire, *while passing urine*).

Aggravation: Evening and morning: After a meal: From motion: In hot weather: After fruit: *From drinking lager beer: During typhoid fever: After abuse of opium* (general condition).

Before Stool: Strong urging: Rumbling: Colic.

During Stool: Smarting and cutting in the anus: Burning in the anus: Colic: Prolapsus ani: Much flatus.

After Stool: Burning in the anus: Intolerable itching, tenderness and soreness of the anus: *Protrusion of dark, purple varices*, somewhat relieved by application of warm water; *much worse from bathing with cold water.*

Accompaniments: Taciturnity or ill-humor. Face suddenly flushing or pale and sunken. *Tongue heavy, like lead, preventing talking;* **shriveled and dry,** *or covered with deep bluish ulcers having black bases.* Dryness of the mouth. Aphthous ulcers in the mouth. Fetid breath. Salivary glands tender and swollen. Aversion to meat. Nausea and vomiting. Stomach will neither tolerate nor digest food; this gastric weakness is most marked about 10 or 11 A. M. *Prolapsus ani during stool and during urination.* Sleepiness in the daytime, sleeplessness at night, with bland delirium, and **inclination to slide down in the bed.** Great debility. *The lower jaw hangs down.*

Perspiration during the first sleep before midnight, with desire to uncover.

Pulse weak and slow, intermitting every third beat. Muscular weakness after abuse of narcotics, soothing syrups, etc.

To delineate **Mur. ac.** further would be to give its full indications in typhoid fever, of which the diarrhœa is only an accompanying symptom. It is also highly applicable to diarrhœa with protrusion of blue or dark purple hæmorrhoids, especially when occurring in feeble children, suffering from gastric atony, muscular debility and threatened marasmus. It follows well after **Rhus.**, or **Bry.**

94. NATRUM CARBONICUM.

Stools: Yellow, fecal; Fecal; Watery or liquid; Thick mucous; Latter part tinged with blood; Expelled with a gush (watery or liquid stool); Sour-smelling.

Aggravation: *After taking milk:* After eating: After taking cold: During a thunder-shower: After vegetables and starchy food (stomach symptoms).

Amelioration: After eating (stomach symptoms).

Before Stool: Cutting: Strong urging: Severe colic, with rumbling in the abdomen.

During Stool: Tenesmus: Burning at the anus.

After Stool: Pain in the rectum.

Accompaniments: Ill-humor. Depression of spirits. Much thirst. Bitter taste of food.

Aversion to milk. Sour eructations. Gnawing and pressure in the stomach, with distension and gone, weak feeling about 10 or 11 A. M.; relieved by eating. Accumulation of wind in the abdomen. Passing much sour or fetid flatus. Griping colic soon after eating. Stitches in the left hypochondrium, worse after drinking very cold water. Weak ankles.

Natr. carb. is rarely indicated in the treatment of diarrhœa, but as one of the remedies having an aggravation from milk, it may sometimes be required in chronic cases. The stomach symptoms should also correspond.

95. NATRUM MURIATICUM.

Stools: *Black, watery; Greenish, watery; Grayish; Like the white of an egg* (without fæces); Bloody;

Profuse; Gushing; Corrosive; Involuntary; Alternating with constipation.

Aggravation: During the day: *After farinaceous food:* In hot weather: By motion.

Before Stool: Rumbling in the abdomen. Wants to pass wind, but knows not whether fæces or wind escapes.

After Stool: Weakness.

Accompaniments: *Sad and enjoys the sadness. Angry when consoled.* Likes to brood over past troubles. Child is irritable and cross when spoken to. Throbbing headache. Face pale, *shining*, *greasy-looking*. Upper lip swollen. *Mapped tongue. Vesicles and herpes about the mouth.* Corners of mouth sore, cracked and crusty. Aphthæ. Scorbutic gums. Child is slow in learning to talk, on account of imperfect development of the muscles of the tongue and larynx. Craving appetite. *Aversion to bread; to coffee. Longing for salt, salt-fish, oysters or bitter things. Loss of taste. Violent thirst, with dry, sticky mouth; worse in the evening.* Nausea and vomiting. Distress in the stomach, relieved by tightening the clothes. Abdomen distended with flatus or sunken. Urine deposits a reddish sediment; passed involuntarily at night and when coughing, walking or laughing. *Severe backache, relieved by pressure and by lying on the back.* Drowsiness, with inability to sleep. Sleep restless, disturbed by dreams. Dreams that robbers are in the house. Ankles weak and turn easily. Swelling of the glands. **General emaciation, most conspicuous about the neck, which is very thin and shrunken.**

Natrum mur. is chiefly useful for chronic diarrhœa of children, but also of older people.

The emaciation of the neck, the greasy appearance of the face and the peculiar desires and aversions furnish the leading indications.

96. NATRUM SULPHURICUM.

Stools: *Thin, yellow fluid;* Half liquid; *Yellowish-green; Gushing;* Spattering all over the vessel; Suddenly expelled; Slimy, light red, or bloody; Involuntary, while passing flatus or urine;

Not frequent; Often painless.

Aggravation: *In the morning (after rising and moving about):* Hereditary in old women:

During the day: After farinaceous food: After a protracted spell of damp weather: From living in damp houses: From cold evening air.

Amelioration: After breakfast and in the open air (general condition).

Before Stool: Contractive pain in the abdomen, extending into the chest: Pinching: Pains in the groins and hypogastrium: *Violent colic and rumbling*.

During Stool: Slight tenesmus and burning in the anus: *Profuse emission of flatus*.

After Stool: Cheerfulness: Happy mood: Burning at the anus: *Relief of colic*.

Accompaniments: *Thirst in the evening*. Sour risings, with heartburn. Bitter taste. Copious formation of gas, causing distension of abdomen and flatulent colic. *Incarceration of flatus* at night, causing great pain, especially in right side. Colic is particularly worse before breakfast when the stomach is empty; relieved by kneading the abdomen and by borborygmus. Bruised pain in the intestines. *Stitches in the region of the liver, and sensitiveness when walking in the open air. Liver is swollen and sore to the touch or to any jar of the body.* Constant uneasiness in the bowels and urging to stool. *Passing of large* *quantities of flatus, mostly fetid.* Constant desire to take a deep, long breath.

Panaritium. Inflammation and suppuration around the roots of the nails. The pain is better out of doors.

Natr. sulph. is one of the most frequently indicated remedies in cases of chronic diarrhœa, where the loose morning stool is the leading symptom. The flatulent symptoms are very characteristic, but not necessarily present.

The tendency to "run rounds," or painful suppurations around the finger-nails, is often present, and is a strong confirmatory indication. The morning stool differs from that of **Sulph.** in occurring later and after rising.

97. NICCOLUM.

Stools: Thin, fecal; Yellow, mucous;
Coming out with force (yellow mucous).

Aggravation: *After taking milk:* In the morning.

Before Stool: Urging: Pinching: Violent cutting in abdomen.

During Stool: Violent burning in anus: Stinging in the rectum: Violent urging: Tenesmus.

After Stool: Colic: Violent burning in anus as if grains of barley were sticking there: Renewed unsuccessful urging and tenesmus.

Accompaniments: Hunger, without appetite

or any relish for food, but feels better after eating.

Much thirst day and night. Nausea, with gulping up of sour water. Distended abdomen.

Much flatulence, fetid or inodorous.

This remedy resembles several others in the aggravation after milk, but differs from them all in other symptoms. We have had no clinical experience with it as yet.

98. NITRIC ACID.

Stools: Mucous; *Green mucous;* Bloody mucous; Slimy; *Flakes of false membranes;* Undigested; Yellowish-white, fluid; *Putrid; Fetid;* Acrid; *Sour-smelling*.

Aggravation: On alternate days: During typhoid fever: After dinner: After milk: After abuse of mercury: *In the morning:* In dark-complexioned old people.

Amelioration: *From riding in a carriage* (general condition): From moving about and eating (nausea).

Before Stool: *Colic:* Drawing pains: Cuttings: Constant pressing in the rectum.

During Stool: Nausea: Colic: Tenesmus: Spasmodic contraction of the anus: Cutting in the anus and rectum.

After Stool: *Exhaustion:* Irritation, anxiety and general uneasiness: Soreness and rawness of of the anus: Burning in the anus: *Violent cutting* *and drawing pains in the rectum, continuing for hours.*

Accompaniments: Irritability or despondency. Anxiety about the disease. Vanishing of thought. Dulness of the head. Headache, aggravated by the jar and rat le of carriages on the street. Pale, yellowish complexion. Ulcers in the mouth and fauces. Ulcers and blisters on the lips. Scorbutic gums. Dryness of the throat. Copious flow of saliva. Putrid smell from the mouth. Sour or bitter taste after eating. Aversion to boiled meat; to sweet things; to bread. Appetite for herring; fat food; earth, chalk, lime, starch. Much thirst, especially in the morning. Cutting in the abdomen (in the morning in bed). Much flatulence and rumbling. Urine dark, with a strong smell, or sourish smell, like the urine of horses. Cold feet (with colic).

Night-sweat. Debility. Intermittent pulse.

Emaciation, especially of the upper arms and thighs. Enlargement of the glands.

According to the published symptoms, **Nitr. ac.** resembles **Alumina,** but those symptoms are not confirmed by clinical observation. The appetite for chalk, lime and similar substances obstinately refuses to yield to this remedy, and we are glad to notice that this symptom is not found in Hahnemann's proving. As one of the remedies having green mucous stools, it should be studied in infantile diarrhœa, particularly after abuse of mercury, or in children of syphilitic parents. It has also proved serviceable in dysentery of a typhoid type, with diphtheritic deposit on the mucous membrane of the intestines. Compare with **Hep.** and **Mezer.** after abuse of **Merc.**

99. NUPHAR LUTEUM.

Stools: Yellow, watery; Fetid; Painless.

Aggravation: *From 4 to 7 A. M.*: In the evening (weakness of the limbs): *During typhoid fever*.

Before stool: Colic (or absence of pain).

After Stool: Relief of colic: Smarting and burning in the anus.

Accompaniments: Great impatience at the slightest contradiction.

Pale face, with discolored eyes.

Sweetish taste in the mouth.

Pricking pains in the rectum as from needles.

Weakness of the sexual organs.

Sensation of weakness and loss of power in the limbs, worse in the evening.

General exhaustion.

Nuphar is not a remedy of wide range. The early morning stool, the weakness of the limbs and the general exhaustion are the leading symptoms.

100. NUX MOSCHATA.

Stools: *Thin, yellow* (like beaten or stirred eggs); Bloody; *Undigested;* Watery; Slimy; Putrid; *Profuse*.

Aggravation: In children (girls?): In persons who take cold easily: *At night:* During dentition: From taking cold: From wetting the feet: *In cool, damp weather:* After milk: After boiled milk: After cold drinks: In the morning: During typhoid fever: During pregnancy:

After eating and drinking (colic):

When riding (nausea).

Amelioration: *By application of moist heat (pains):* By lying extended on the back.

Before Stool: Cuttings.

During Stool: Urging.

After Stool: Acrid feeling in the anus: Sensation as if more stool would pass: *Drowsiness.*

Accompaniments: Fitful mood. Inclination to laugh. Sluggish flow of ideas. *Mouth very dry.* Saliva like cotton. Dryness of the mouth, with taste as after eating strongly salted food. Chalky, or pappy taste. Little or no thirst. Craving hunger, or loss of appetite after a few mouthfuls. *Enormous distension of the abdomen after each meal. Feeling as though the food formed itself into lumps with hard surfaces and angles, which cause soreness in the stomach. The dyspeptic symptoms come on while the patient is still at the table.* Nausea, more while riding. Colic, worse after taking food or drink, *relieved by hot, wet cloths.* Urine scanty.

Great drowsiness. *Torpor. Lethargy.*

Cool, dry skin. **Disposition to faint.**

Great languor.

In the exhausting diarrhœas of children, accompanied by great sleepiness, and worse at night, **Nux mosch.** is the remedy.

101. NUX VOMICA.

Stools: *Thin, brownish, mucous; Thin, bloody, mucous;* Thin, green, mucous; *Dark, thin, fecal;* Dark, watery; Brown, fluid; Alternating with constipation;

Frequent; Small; Corrosive; Offensive; Involuntary.

Aggravation: *After debauchery: After abuse of alcoholic spirits: After drastic medicines or prolonged drugging: After change of food (infants):* After night-watching: During jaundice: After taking cold: *In the morning* (general condition): After over-exertion of the mind: After anger: After ginger or brandy (pains): During the day.

Before Stool: Cutting about the umbilicus: *Backache, as if broken: Constant urging (often ineffectual).*

During Stool: Cutting: *Backache: Violent tenesmus.*

After Stool: *Cessation of the pains and tenesmus:* Burning at the anus: *Sensation as if more stool would pass.*

Accompaniments: Irritability. *Over-sensitiveness to external impressions, light, noise, strong smells, jar, etc.* Dull headache. Yellowness of the eyes and face. Pale, earthy color of the face.

Gums swollen, bleeding. Bad smell from the mouth. Tongue coated thick, dirty yellowish-white. *Thirst.* Loss of appetite. Aversion to bread, coffee, tobacco, ale. Desire for chalk, brandy, *fat food.* Putrid, sour or bitter taste. Hiccough. Nausea, in the morning and after dinner. Intolerance of the pressure of the clothing about the hypochondria.

Colic: pinching, cutting, contractive, griping.

Pain, as if the contents of the abdomen were sore and raw. Much flatulence.

Painful, ineffectual desire to urinate.

Frequent urging to urinate.

Drowsiness in the daytime and after eating. *Wakes at 2 or 3 A. M. and lies awake for an hour or two, then falls into a heavy sleep and awakens late in the morning, feeling tired and unrefreshed.*

Debility. Sinking at the stomach. *Desire to sit or lie down.* Sensitiveness to open air, or to a slight current of air. **Heat, with red face and aversion to uncovering.**

Emaciation. Chlorosis.

Nux vom. is often of first importance in dysentery, with the characteristic stools and immediate accompaniments. In slow fevers, with alternating constipation and diarrhœa, and in chlorosis, as well as jaundice, it holds an important place. In the latter affections the general symptoms, more than the stools, decide for this remedy.

Nux must not be overlooked in the treatment of diarrhœa because more often used for constipation.

102. OLEANDER.

Stools: Thin, yellow, fecal; *Undigested (food of the previous day);* Watery; Sour; Frequent; Scanty; *Involuntary (when emitting flatus).*

Aggravation: In the morning: In children.

Before Stool: Rumbling in the abdomen: *Burning in anus.*

After Stool: Burning in anus.

Accompaniments: Pale, sunken face in the morning, with blue rings around the eyes. Canine hunger, and hasty eating without appetite. Thirst for cold water. White-coated tongue. Aversion to cheese. Nausea and vomiting; of mucus; of sour, liquid food; of yellowish green, bitter water. After vomiting, ravenous hunger and thirst.

Rolling and rumbling in the intestines, with emission of much flatulence; of fetid flatulence like rotten eggs.

Some children are much troubled with frequent soiling of the clothes when passing flatus. **Oleander** cures this, and also more acute attacks of involuntary and of indigested stools, as described above.

It has also been found useful in the diarrhœa of tuberculous patients.

103. OPIUM.

Stools: Watery; Dark, fluid, frothy; *Offensive; Involuntary.*

Aggravation: *After fright:* After sudden joy· *During typhoid fever.*

During Stool: Burning in the anus: Tenesmus.

Accompaniments: *Drowsiness or sopor. Sopor, without vomiting or stool.* Apathy. *Stupid, comatose sleep, with rattling, snoring breathing,* or slumber with half-open eyes, *contracted or sluggish pupils*, carphologia, and touching surrounding objects. Muttering delirium. Stupid sleepiness, with frightful visions. *Sleepy, but cannot sleep*. Face bloated, *dark red and hot*, or pale, clay-colored and sunken. Dryness of the mouth. Aversion to food. Nausea.

Urine scanty, retained or suppressed. *Slow, full pulse*.

Profuse sweat.

Convulsions; on entering the fit, loud screams, as from fright; after the fit, sopor.

Fainting, worse on rising. Rapid emaciation.

Opium is chiefly useful in diarrhœa during typhoid fever, but also sometimes indicated in the last stage of infantile diarrhœa, with the characteristic stools and convulsions.

104. OXALIC ACID.

Stools: Muddy, brown, fecal; Watery; Mucous and bloody;

Involuntary (a constant discharge, white mucous).

Aggravation: *After coffee: In the morning: After breakfast:* When lying down:

From motion: From eating sugar (pains).

Amelioration: From rest (pains).

Before Stool: Headache: Twisting colic around the navel.

During Stool: Colic about the navel: Colicky pains seem to radiate from a small spot. Violent urging: Griping pains in the anus so severe as to cause headache and heat in the head.

After Stool: Nausea: Relief of pain in small of back: Dryness of the throat: Cramps in the calves.

Accompaniments: *Thinking of the symptoms aggravates them.* Exhilaration.

Stomach very sensitive to pressure.

Frequent pains and soreness about the navel. Copious urine.

105. PAULLINIA SORBILIS.

(Guarana.)

Stools: *Green, odorless, mucous; Profuse;* Bloody with bright green flakes.

Aggravation: During dentition: In summer.

Accompaniments: Loss of appetite.

Restlessness.

Sleeplessness.

Although **Paullinia** has been before the profession over twenty years, since its introduction by the Vienna provers, the concomitants are still almost unknown. The peculiar stool, however, has often been verified in practice and must always furnish the leading indication for the use of this remedy in infantile diarrhœa.

106. PETROLEUM.

Stools: *Yellowish, watery;* Brownish-yellow, pasty; Brown, watery; Bloody mucous; Watery and bloody, containing scrapings of the intestines;

Mucous; Green, slimy;

Profuse; *Gushing*.

Aggravation: After deranging the stomach: *After saur-kraut: After cabbage:* After riding in a carriage: During pregnancy: Waking one in the morning: During stormy weather: *Always in the daytime*.

Amelioration: By bending double (colic): By eating (pains in the stomach).

Before Stool: Colic: Cutting and pinching: Sudden urging.

During Stool: Colic: Tenesmus.

After Stool: Great weakness and dizziness:

Canine hunger: Urging: Much pressing as if large quantities were yet to be expelled.

Accompaniments: Ill-humor. Vehemence. *Pulsating occipital headache* in the morning. White-coated tongue. Fetid smell from the mouth. Saliva smells badly. Smell from the mouth like onions, or putrid, slimy mouth. Bitter or sour taste. Aversion to meat; fat food; and warm, cooked food. Nausea and vomiting: in the morning; when riding in a carriage.

Cold feeling in the abdomen. Distension of abdomen, with much offensive flatus. *Feeling of great emptiness in the stomach, as after long fasting. Weak, empty feeling in the bowels.* Gastralgia, with drawing, pressing pains, relieved by eating.

Pinching colic, arousing one from sleep toward morning, relieved by bending double. *Canine hunger after stool*, quickly satisfied. Exhaustion. Drowsiness. Emaciation. Aversion to the open air, which causes chilliness.

Restless sleep, the patient waking often, and *imagining that other persons lie in the same bed*, or speaking of himself in the third person.

The most striking symptom of **Petr.** is the last one mentioned above, and one that often indicates this remedy in delirious states accompanying diarrhœa (or other affections). If unable to complete the cure, it will produce a favorable change and prepare the way for some other remedy.

It is also useful in chronic diarrhœa with the aggravations and other symptoms as given above.

107. PHOSPHORUS.

Stools: *Green mucous;* Greenish, turning blue on standing, White, mucous; *White watery; Green watery;* Yellow watery; Bilious; Bluish; Watery, with lumps of white mucus, or *little grains like tallow; Undigested; Bloody;* Brown, fluid; *Bloody and purulent;* **Oozing from the constantly open anus** (*green and bloody*)*; Bloody water, like the washings of meat; Profuse;* Alternating with constipation;

Hot; Involuntary (on the least motion; when coughing); *Passing out with force; Pouring out as from a hydrant;*

Fetid; Sour-smelling; Corrosive; Painless.

Aggravation: *In the morning:* Day and night: In lean, slender persons: *From lying on the left side: From warm food: After eating or nursing:* In childbed: During pregnancy: During cholera time.

Amelioration: **After cold food, ice or ice-cream** (*symptoms of the stomach*): *After sleeping* (*general condition*): From lying on the right side.

Before Stool: Rumbling: Colic: Heat or chilliness: Sudden urging.

During Stool: Smarting in the rectum: Protrusion of hæmorrhoids and sharp, stitching pain from coccyx to inter-scapular region, and even to the vertex.

After Stool: Burning at the anus: Tenesmus: Empty feeling in the abdomen: Weakness, obliging one to lie down: Exhaustion: Fainting.

Accompaniments: Excitability. Vehemence. Pale, sallow or changeable color of the face, with sunken eyes and blue rings around them. Tongue dry; white; clean; moist and cracked. Red, dry streak down the middle of the tongue. Canine hunger at night, with great weakness if not gratified. Loss of appetite. *Thirst, with desire for very cold drinks*, especially at night, for something refreshing. Taste sweetish; saltish; sour; bitter after eating. *Vomiting of what has* *been drunk* as soon as it has become warm in the stomach. **Vomiting relieved for a time by ice or very cold food or drink.** Burning in the stomach. Heartburn. Rising up of hot, sour ingesta. Abdomen swollen. **Weak, gone feeling in the abdomen,** *with burning between the shoulders.* Abdomen very sensitive, painful to touch. Rolling and rumbling in abdomen during and after drinking. Fetid flatus. **Anus constantly open.** Burning of the palms of the hands.

Profuse, pale, watery urine.

Emaciation. Nervous debility. Over-sensitiveness of all the senses. *Sleepiness in the daytime and after meals.* Sleeplessness before midnight. Frequent waking, with feeling of great heat. Profuse night-sweats. Glandular swellings.

The stools of **Phos.** are hardly characteristic unless the little grains of tallow (they resemble more opaque frog spawn, or sago, as I have seen them) should prove to be so. The condition and accompaniments are, however, very peculiar, and are also constant. They will always be present in more or less completeness when this remedy is indicated, and will render a brilliant cure almost certain if the remedy is given in a proper dose, and is not repeated after the improvement has fully begun.

The symptoms of **Phos.** are most frequently met with in chronic cases. It is often well to give a single dose of a high potency of **Nux vom.** a few hours before beginning with **Phos.**, particularly in cases coming from allopathic treatment.

108. PHOSPHORIC ACID.

Stools: *Whitish watery; Yellow, watery, with meal-like sediment;* Light, yellow, fecal; Whitish-gray, fecal; *Undigested;* Greenish-white mucous; Like dirty white paint;

Involuntary (while passing flatus);

Painless; Very offensive.

Aggravation: During typhoid fever: *From depressing mental emotions:* After taking acids: After loss of animal fluids: *In young persons who have grown very rapidly:* Night and morning: *After eating:* Lying on right side.

During Stool: Profuse emission of flatus.

Accompaniments: Indifference. Quiet delirium and stupefaction. Somnolency. Complexion pale, sickly. Glassy appearance of the eyes. Scrobutic gums, swollen, readily bleeding. Tongue covered with gluey mucus. Voracious appetite. Much thirst. *Desire for something refreshing or juicy.* Dryness of the mouth, with viscid, frothy, tenacious mucus. Abdomen bloated. Much fermentation in the bowels, with rumbling and gurgling of flatus. Frequent emission of pale, watery urine, forming a white cloud at once, or opaque and milky when passed.

Profuse perspiration at night.

Cramps of upper arm, forearm and wrists.

Phos. ac. is one of the most prominent remedies for white or yellow watery diarrhœa, either chronic or acute. It is characterized by painlessness and the absence of any marked debility or exhaustion, the patient even gaining flesh in spite of the diarrhœa.

109. PICRIC ACID.

Stools: Thin, yellow, oily; Yellowish-gray (like gruel).

Aggravation: After mental exertion (headache and burning in spine): On awaking (backache): In the evening (general condition).

During Stool: Burning, smarting and cutting at the anus.

After Stool: Great prostration: Burning and smarting of the anus.

Accompaniments: Great indifference. *Lack of will-power to undertake any work.* Dull pressive headache in forehead or occiput. Any attempt to use the mind brings on the headache and causes *burning along the spine*. Pupils dilated. Bitter taste, with thirst. Sour eructations. Nausea, worse in the morning and on attempting to rise and move about. Pressure in the stomach, with desire to belch. Rumbling of flatus in the abdomen. Tendency to jaundice.

Legs feel heavy like lead. Weakness of the legs and back, with soreness of the muscles and joints. Heat in lower part of spine; tired aching in lumbar region on awaking. *Restless sleep, with priapismic erections.* General sense of lassitude. The least exertion causes prostration. *Feet cold. Chilliness followed by clammy sweat. Great feeling of fatigue.*

Picric acid presents a perfect picture of "brain-fag," and although not well defined as a remedy for acute diseases of the bowels, ought to prove serviceable in diarrhœa occurring in persons exhausted by mental overwork.

110. PLANTAGO.

Stools: *Brown, fermented, frothy; Watery, brown;* Watery; Papescent; Excoriating (watery, brown stools).

Aggravation: From 8 to 10 A. M.

Amelioration: By eating (colic): By motion (general condition).

Before Stool: Colic: Frequent discharge of offensive flatus.

During Stool: Violent griping pains, with tenesmus (or absence of pain): Partial prolapse of rectum: Weakness: Faintness.

Accompaniments: Irritability. Despondency. Confusion of thought. Dull headache. Tongue coated white, with dirty, putrid or clammy taste. Gums bleed easily. Fetid breath. Appetite poor. Thirst. Eructations tasting like sulphur or carbonic acid gas. Nausea, with drowsiness or faint tremulous feeling. Sinking feeling at the stomach. Distension of abdomen, with frequent loud and copious discharge of fetid flatus.

Rumbling and uneasiness in the bowels. Violent griping pains, mostly in the upper part of the abdomen. Sensation of goneness in the abdomen. *Frequent and profuse discharge of colorless urine. Nocturnal, copious enuresis from laxity of sphincter vesicæ.* Grinding of the teeth during sleep. Sleep restless, disturbed by dreams.

Weariness and prostration, with desire to yawn and stretch.

The colic, relieved by eating, and the urinary symptoms will distinguish **Plantago** from other remedies having similar stools.

111. PLUMBUM METALLICUM.

Stools: *Watery, dark, offensive;* Yellow; Mucous and bloody; Bloody; Profuse (watery stools); Involuntary.

Before Stool: Frequent and almost fruitless urging: Violent constriction of the anus.

During Stool: Tenesmus: Violent tearing in the anus.

After Stool: Tenesmus.

Accompaniments: *Delirium alternating with the colic.* Face pale or sallow. Nausea and vomiting. Severe cutting pains in the abdomen, extorting violent screams: these pains may radiate to the brain, causing delirium; or to the lungs, producing dyspnœa; or to other parts of the body. *Constriction and retraction of the abdomen.* **Sensation of something pulling at the umbilicus, with actual retraction of the navel.**

Plumbum is rarely indicated, but has proved curative in both diarrhœa and dysentery, when the above italicized symptoms were present.

112. PODOPHYLLUM.

Stools: *Watery, with meal-like sediment; Yellow, pasty;* Black; *Yellow, watery;* Like dirty water; Greenish slimy;

Greenish watery; Dark yellow, mucous;

Jelly-like, mucous; White, slimy, mucous; *Bloody and green mucous; Mucous and blood-streaked;*

Chalk-like, fecal; Undigested; Changeable; Frothy;

Involuntary (during sleep and when passing flatus);

Profuse, frequent, gushing, painless (watery stools);

Very offensive, like carrion (yellow, mucous stools).

Aggravation: *In the morning: In the night: During hot weather:* After taking milk and acid fruit together: After eating or drinking: During dentition: Lying on the back (colic): While being washed.

Amelioration: By bending double, lying on the side, by pressure of the hands on the abdomen, and by warmth (colic).

Before Stool: Sudden urging: Loud gurgling, as of water: *Violent colic (or absence of pain): Prolapsus ani.*

During Stool: *Prolapsus ani: Colic (or absence of pain): Pains in the sacrum:* Emission of flatus: Tenesmus (dysenteric stools).

After Stool: *Prolapsus ani: Exhaustion:* Flushes of heat up the back: Colic continues: Sense of weakness in the abdomen and rectum: Soreness of the anus.

Accompaniments: Headache, alternating with diarrhœa. *Rolling of the head during dentition.* Perspiration on the head, with coldness of the flesh during dentition. Bad smell from the mouth (at night). Tongue coated yellowish or white. Tongue dry. Loss of appetite. Violent thirst or thirstlessness. Desire for acids. Sour regurgitation of food. Acid eructations. Vomiting: hot; of food; of bile; of frothy green mucus. *Gagging or empty retching.* Colic, with retraction of the abdominal muscles. Transient abdominal pains, relieved by pressure. Sinking feeling at the epigastrium, with sensation as if everything would drop through the pelvis. Heat in the bowels. Suppression of urine. Sleepiness in the daytime, more in the forenoon. Restless sleep, with half-closed eyes, moaning, grinding of the teeth. Great restlessness, tossing about the bed, yawning and stretching, with entire relief while doing so. Cold, clammy skin.

Softness of the flesh, with debility.

Sallowness of the skin. Jaundice. Dark brown urine.

Violent cramps of the feet, calves and thighs

(with painless watery stools), *with yawning and stretching*.

There is no remedy so surely indicated by painless cholera morbus as **Podoph.** The stools are profuse and gushing, each seeming to drain the patient dry, but soon he is full again. There may also be violent cramps. It would seem that it must prove to be similar to many cases of cholera, but clinical experience in this direction is still wanting. We hope that some of our colleagues, who have the opportunity, will test it in this fearful scourge. In diarrhœas of infants it ranks also among the first to be referred to. It resembles **Calc. c.** and **Phos. ac.**, yet can easily be distinguished from the former by careful attention to the concomitant symptoms, and from the latter by the more rapid debility and exhaustion.

113. PSORINUM.

Stools: *Dark brown, thin, fluid; Black, watery;* Green mucous, mixed with blood;

Very offensive, like rotten eggs;

Frequent; Involuntary; Nearly painless.

Aggravation: *During dentition: After severe, acute disease: At night: Early in the morning:* When rising in the morning: In childbed: When the weather changes (general condition): With east winds.

Before Stool: Griping pains about the navel.
Accompaniments: Excitable, anxious. *Utter*

hopelessness during convalescence. Child constantly fretting and worrying; nervous, cries out at night. Face pale, sickly-looking, emaciated. Eructations smelling like rotten eggs. *Canine hunger*, even after a hearty meal and at night. *Canine hunger preceding the attacks.* Loss of appetite during convalescence. Desire for acids. Deep-seated, heavy pain in the region of the liver, worse from pressure, lying on it, coughing, laughing, or on deep inspiration.

Emission of fetid, sulphurous flatulence. Soft stool is discharged with difficulty. Sleepiness in the daytime. *Great debility. Profuse perspiration from the least exertion at night.* Restless sleep; awakens terrified. **Skin dirty, greasy looking,** *with yellow blotches here and there, and a partially developed eruption on the forehead and chest.*

Body always has a filthy smell, even after a bath. Feels particularly well the day before an attack.

Sick babies will not sleep day or night, but worry, fret and cry.

Although the dark fluid stool is very characteristic of **Psor.,** the very offensive odor is much more so. This alone often indicates it in infantile diarrhœa, or in cholera infantum, whatever may be the stool; and it will usually produce a favorable change at once, and often complete the cure. It is also valuable as an intercurrent, when well-chosen remedies fail to relieve, here rivaling **Sulph.** Whether derived from purest gold or purest filth, our gratitude for its excellent services forbids us to inquire or care.

114. PULSATILLA.

Stools: *Greenish, bilious, watery;* Yellow, mucous, mixed with blood; White and bloody mucous; *Green, mucous;* Changeable; Frequent; Scanty; Purulent;

Offensive; Corrosive; Involuntary (during sleep at night); Clear yellow red or green slime.

Aggravation: *At night:* After measles: After pork or fat food: *After ice-cream: After fruit* (strawberries?): After tobacco: After cold drinks: From damp places: **From warmth or in a warm room** (general condition): During cholera time.

Amelioration: *In the open air or a cool place* (general condition).

Before Stool: *Rumbling: Cutting colic: Pains in the small of the back.*

During Stool: *Shaking chill:* Pain in the small of the back.

After Stool: Colic, as from flatulence: *Chilliness* in the small of the back: Smarting of the anus: Tenesmus from the anus up along the sacrum.

Accompaniments: Peevishness or *weeping mood*. Weeps when telling her symptoms. Vertigo after eating or stooping. Pale, bloated face, with sunken eyes. Burning of the right cheek. Tongue coated white. Great sensation of dryness in the mouth, without thirst. Bad smell from the mouth. Increase of saliva. Tenacious mucus in the mouth. *Constant spitting* of frothy, cotton-like mucus. *Bitter taste in the mouth, and after food or drink.* Putrid taste. *Thirstlessness*, or thirst for ale, lemonade or spirits. *Loss of taste.* Aversion to fat; to meat; to bread; to milk.

Vomiting of food; of bile; of mucus; of bitter or *sour* fluid.

Flatulent colic. Painful rumbling of flatulence. Passage of fetid flatus. Difficulty of breathing, worse at night.

Irresistible desire for fresh air.

Chilliness. Chlorosis.

"These kinds of nightly diarrhœa are characteristic of **Pul.**, and there is scarcely a drug which occasions them as often."—HAHNEMANN.

115. RAPHANUS SATIVUS.

Stools: *Brown, or yellow-brown, fluid;* Undigested;

Green liquid, mixed with mucus and blood;

Frothy, copious and passing out with much force (brown, fluid stool).

Aggravation: After taking milk and water (colic): When lying down (nausea): After eating.

Accompaniments: Anguish, with dread of death, which is supposed to be near. Face expressive of pain and exhaustion. Thick, white coating of the tongue. Tongue pale reddish-blue, with deep fissure in the middle. **Bitter taste.**

Violent thirst. Constant nausea, or nausea occurring in paroxysms, with faintness and inability to lie down. Vomiting of food, with white mucus; of bile and water. Vomiting is preceded by shuddering over the back and arms. Colic. *No emission of flatus by mouth or anus for a long time. Protrusion of intestines like pads all over the abdomen, here and there, during the pains.* Urine yellow, turbid, with copious sediment looking like yeast. Great weakness and languor.

Much clinical experience with **Raphanus** has confirmed the symptom, "No emission of flatus by mouth or anus for a long time," as one of priceless value.

116. RHEUM.

Stools: Mucous and fecal; Thin, brownish, fecal; Brown, slimy, mucous; Whitish, curdy, turning green on the diaper on exposure to the air; Fæces mixed with green slime; *Sour-smelling;* Fetid; Frothy; Fermented; Corrosive.

Aggravation: When moving about: In children: In infants: After eating: *During dentition:* In childbed: During inflammatory rheumatism: In hot weather; When uncovered (pains).

Amelioration: By bending double (colic).

Before Stool: *Colic: Urging:* Ineffectual urging to urinate.

During Stool: Colic: Chilliness: Screaming,

with drawing up of the limbs or stiffening of the body.

After Stool: *Tenesmus:* Renewed urging (when moving): Constrictive, cutting colic, worse from any motion (*or relief of colic*).

Accompaniments: Restlessness. Demanding various things with vehemence and crying. Pale face. Cool perspiration on the face, especially around the nose and mouth. *Desire for various kinds of food, which become repugnant as soon as a little is eaten.* Nausea. Salivation. Cutting colic, relieved by bending double and much worse when standing. Liver-colored, dark, smarting urine. Dysuria. Restless sleep, with tossing, crying out and *twitchings of the muscles of the face and hands.*

Sour smell of the whole body.

The sour-smelling stool has always been regarded as the most characteristic symptom of **Rheum**. It is not one of the most frequently indicated remedies, and still less so on account of its constant abuse allopathically.

"May be given after abuse of Magnesia, *with or without rhubarb*, if stools are sour."—H. N. GUERNSEY.

117. RHODODENDRON.

Stools: Thin, brownish, fecal; Undigested; Spurting out with force.

Aggravation: *In cold, damp weather:* During

or before a thunder-shower: After meals: *After fruit:*

On rising from the bed: When walking (nausea).

Accompaniments: Indifference and aversion to all occupation. Rumbling in the abdomen and discharge of fetid flatus. Sinking at the stomach. Nausea. *General rheumatic pains, brought on by damp, cold weather, and worse during wet.*

The aggravations distinguish **Rhodod.**

118. RHUS TOXICODENDRON.

Stools: Dark yellow, watery; *Thin, red, mucous; Thin, yellow, mucous; Bloody; Jelly-like mucous,* streaked white and yellow; Greenish, mucous, with jelly-like globules or flakes; Mucous, bloody and slimy; *Lumps of transparent mucus;* **Bloody water, like washings of beef;** Yellowish-white, fecal;

Yellow, fluid; Dark red (brick-colored) fluid; Otter-colored fluid (typhoid); *Profuse* (yellow, watery stools); *Scanty, frequent* (bloody water); Alternating with constipation;

Involuntary (at night while sleeping); *Fetid;* Frothy and *painless* (yellow fluid); *Very offensive* (dark yellow, watery); *Odorless* (*bloody watery; yellow fluid*).

Aggravation: *During typhoid fever:* After drinking ice-water: *After getting wet:* In cool, damp weather: After excessive bodily exercise: *After a strain:* At night.

Amelioration: When bending double, and when lying on the abdomen (colic); From warmth and *continued motion* (general condition).

Before Stool: Constant urging, with nausea and tearing colic: Cutting colic.

During Stool: Cutting colic: Urging: *Nausea: Tenesmus:* **Tearing pains down the thighs.**

After Stool: *Remission of the pains and urging:* Pains leave the abdomen and go to sacrum, and then extend down the posterior part of thighs to heels: Must keep legs in motion, which relieves: Feeling of great weight in rectum:
Tenesmus.

Accompaniments: Headache. *Restlessness.* Loquacious delirium. Feels as if sinking through the bed. Pale, sunken face, with blue rings around the eyes. Putrid taste and smell from the mouth. Lips dry, brown or black. *Tongue dry and rough, with* **red edges and triangular red tip;** coated dirty white, yellow or brown; or *clean, red and cracked.* Increase of saliva. Bitter taste of food, especially bread. Metallic taste. Loss of appetite. Desire for oysters. *Much thirst*, more at night, arising mostly from dryness of the mouth. Thirst for cold water; *for cold milk. Nausea.*

Cutting, tearing and pinching colic. *Fermentation in the abdomen.*

Pains in all the limbs. *Tearing pains down the*

thighs. Has to change position often to get relief.

Restless sleep. Comatose sleep. *Troublesome dreams, vivid, of hard work and difficulty.*

The stools of **Rhus tox.** are quite characteristic, and many of the conditions and accompaniments are very much so. It is frequently applicable in dysentery, mostly after other remedies, and in a late stage, when the disease shows a tendency to assume a typhoid type. The craving for cold milk and the laborious dreams of excessive bodily exertion, as running, wading in the snow, hurrying, and the like, are more characteristic of this remedy than of any other. It has been observed that **Rhus tox.** and **Apis m.** do not follow each other well.

119. RUMEX CRISPUS.

Stools: *Brownish, watery; Thin, brownish, fecal;* Offensive; Generally painless; Profuse.

Aggravation: *In the morning (before rising):* From moving (nausea).

Before Stool: Sudden urging, driving one out of bed: Nausea: Colic.

Accompaniments: Severe headache. Mouth dry. Tongue coated yellow. Nausea and eructations.

Violent dry cough, excited by tickling in the larynx, often almost continuous, worse at night; when walking; when inhaling cool air; when talking; by pressure on the larynx or trachea; when lying on the left side. Much debility.

The chief application of **Rumex** is to cases having the characteristic cough accompanying the diarrhœa. It has also proved useful, however, in morning diarrhœa where **Sulph.** seemed indicated, but did not cure.

120. SABADILLA.

Stools: *Brown, fermented, swimming on the water;* Liquid, bloody and slimy.

Aggravation: In children: Every fourth day (worm symptoms):

At precisely the same hour (general condition).

Amelioration: By lying down (general condition).

Before Stool: Pinching around the umbilicus: Loud rumbling: Urging:

Emission of flatus.

After Stool: Burning in the abdomen and rectum.

Accompaniments: Headache, produced or aggravated by mental exertion. Tongue sore, coated yellow, with white centre. Taste bitter, sweet or lost. Ptyalism. Aversion to food; to *meat;* to sour things; to coffee; or canine hunger, with desire for sweets and farinaceous food, alternating with disgust for meat, wine and sour things. Sour or rancid eructations. Nausea and desire to vomit. Burning in stomach and along œsophagus, with vomiting, cutting colic, nervous debility and twitchings. Below pit of the stomach feeling of a sore spot on pressure and during inspiration. Spasmodic constriction of the abdominal muscles on the left side, with burning pains. Sensation of a ball moving and turning rapidly in the abdomen. Abdomen bloated. Sensation as if abdomen were sunken. Stitches in the hypochondria. Rumbling in the abdomen, as if empty. Emission of much flatus. *Urine thick and turbid like muddy water.* Cold feet. Drowsy during day, restless at night. Chilliness and sensitiveness to cold.

Sabadilla will occasionally prove useful in the diarrhœa of light-haired children of lax muscular fibre, suffering from verminous affections. It differs from **Cina** and **Stannum** both in the stools and in the concomitants.

121. SAMBUCUS NIGER.

Stools: Thin, slimy; Yellow, fecal; Watery; Frequent.

Aggravation: In scrofulous children.

Before Stool: Urging.

During Stool: Profuse emission of flatus.

After Stool: Renewed urging.

Accompaniments: Nervousness, with tendency to start. Thirst, but drinks are not palatable. Distended abdomen, with pressure and griping in the stomach and umbilical region.

Drowsiness, with inability to sleep. Sleep with mouth and eyes half open. *Dry heat of the body, with coldness of the feet and hands during sleep; on awaking the face breaks out into profuse sweat, which extends over the body and continues more or less during waking hours; on going to sleep again the dry heat returns. No thirst during heat or sweat.* Most of the pains occur during rest and disappear during motion.

The stools of **Samb.** present no special indications; but the dry heat during sleep, breaking out into sweat on awaking, and the absence of thirst, are very characteristic; and when these concomitants are present, **Samb.** will quickly remove the whole train of morbid phenomena.

122. SANGUINARIA CANADENSIS.

Stools: Watery; Thin, fecal; Undigested.

Aggravation: *After coryza and catarrh:* After the pains in the chest.

Before Stool: Severe cutting pains: Urging.

During Stool: Discharge of much flatus.

Accompaniments: Loss of appetite. White-coated tongue. Desire for piquant, highly-seasoned food. *Nausea*, not diminished by vomiting. Vomiting of bitter water. Profuse salivation, with the nausea and vomiting. Craving to eat in order to quiet the nausea. Goneness in the stomach, especially after eating. Frequent discharge of very offensive flatus. Much debility.

The aggravations and the nausea are chiefly characteristic of **Sang. c.**

123. SARSAPARILLA.

Stools: Watery or semi-liquid.

Aggravation: *In the spring:* After washing.

Before Stool: Violent cutting in the abdomen.
During Stool: Profuse emission of flatus.
After Stool: Faintness.

Accompaniments: Face yellow, wrinkled, old looking. *Apthæ on tongue and roof of mouth.* Tongue clean or coated white. Salivation. Taste metallic or nauseous. Good appetite. Absence of thirst. Nausea and vomiting. *Colic and back ache at the same time.* Burning or cold feeling in the abdomen, with sensation of emptiness. Rumbling and fermentation in the abdomen, with discharge of offensive flatus. *Child screams when urinating. Urine deposits white sand. Neck emaciated and shrunken.* Predominant chilliness. *Great emaciation, the skin shriveled and lying in folds.* Small flat warts on the hands. Warts under the ends of the finger-nails.

Sarsaparilla is especially useful for marasmus, following cholera infantum, and after abuse of mercury.

124. SCILLA.

Stools: *Dark brown or black, slimy, fluid, in frothy bubbles;*

Very offensive; Painless; Involuntary (when coughing, sneezing or passing urine).

Aggravation: In the morning (2 to 7 A. M.): During the day: During measles.

Accompaniments: Much viscid mucus in the mouth. Desire for acids. Thirst. Bread tastes bitter. Soup and meat taste sweet. Pressure in the stomach as from a stone. Nausea. Vomiting. Cutting colic. Frequent discharge of very fetid flatus.

Profuse urine.

A very careful comparison will sometimes be necessary in order to distinguish **Scilla** from **Psorinum.** The stools are very similar, but those of **Scilla** are frothy, and there is an absence of the debility which usually accompanies the stools of the other remedy. It is also useful after **Bryonia.**

125. SECALE CORNUTUM.

Stools: *Watery and slimy; Yellowish; Greenish; Olive green;* Brownish; Watery and flocculent; *Colorless*, watery;

Profuse; Frequent; Offensive; Putrid; Fetid; *Gushing; Involuntary; Sudden attack.*

Aggravation: In childbed: After cholera: During typhoid fever:

After eating or drinking (vomiting).

Before Stool: Cutting and rumbling in the abdomen.

During Stool: Cutting: Great exhaustion: Coldness.

After Stool: Great exhaustion.

Accompaniments: Anxiety. Fear of death. Pale and sunken face. Features distorted. Eyes sunken deep in the sockets and surrounded with a blue margin. Dryness of the mouth. Dry, thick, viscid, yellowish-white coating on the tongue. Tongue cold and livid. *Unquenchable thirst.* Desire for sour things; *for lemonade.* Constant nausea, worse after eating. *Much empty retching. Vomiting:* of food; of bile; of mucus; *of green, offensive, watery fluid; painless and without effort, with great weakness. Vomiting immediately after eating. Severe anxiety and burning at the pit of the stomach.* Burning in the abdomen. Frequent rumbling, flatulence and fulness of the abdomen. Colic worse at night. *Suppression of urine.* Voice feeble and inaudible, or hoarse and hollow.

Skin cold, blue, *shriveled.* Coldness in the back, abdomen and limbs, with formication in the back and legs. Cramps in the chest, *hands and toes. Fingers and toes spread apart or bent backward.*

Great debility. *Sudden and great exhaustion.*

Cold, clammy perspiration over the whole body. *Icy coldness of the extremities.* **Aversion to heat, or to being covered.**

Nothing is more characteristic of **Secale** than the aversion to being covered, or to heat. This will often distinguish it from many other remedies that have, otherwise, similar symptoms, especially **Arsen.**, which has desire for heat and covering. It may be distinguished from **Camph.** by the violent thirst, and also by paying attention to the fact that the cold spells of the latter remedy often occur at night, passing off in the morning. The choleraic stool is not offensive, except, perhaps, at first, but that occurring in childbed is so. In cholera morbus it most resembles **Colchicum,** and is followed well by **China.**

126. SEPIA.

Stools: *Green*, mucous; *Green*, slimy, mucous; Jelly-like; Bloody; *Almost constant oozing from the anus;*

Expelled quickly; Frequent; Not profuse; Fetid; Sour; Putrid; Painless.

Aggravation: After milk: *After taking boiled milk: During dentition:* In children: After taking meat: After eating potatoes: During pregnancy: After sea-bathing.

Before Stool: *Nausea:* Colic.

During Stool: Prolapsus ani: Jerking pains from anus upward through the rectum.

After Stool: Exhaustion: Debility: Prolapsus ani.

Accompaniments: Jerking of the head backward and forward. Fontanelles open. Face pale or sallow, yellow about the mouth and yellow saddle across the nose. Eyes sunken. Bad smell from the mouth. Aphthæ. Tongue coated white. Putrid or sour taste. Food tastes too salt. Aversion to meat and milk. Thirst in the morning. Sour or fetid eructations. Nausea. Vomiting. Discharge of much offensive flatus. *Gone feeling in the stomach, not relieved by eating*. Involuntary urination at night in the first sleep. *Urine turbid, offensive, with reddish or clay-colored sedi-*

ment, adhering closely to the vessel. Palms of hands and soles of feet burning hot. Sleepiness in the daytime. Frequent waking at night. Waking at three in the morning and inability to fall asleep again. *Rapid exhaustion and emaciation.*

Sepia fills an important place in the treatment of infantile diarrhœa. The aggravation from boiled milk, and the rapid exhaustion, are distinguishing symptoms. It is also applicable in chronic, debilitating diarrhœa.

127. SILICEA.

Stools: Liquid, slimy, frothy; Mucous; Reddish, mucous; Bloody; Watery; Purulent; Pasty Undigested; Scanty; Frequent;

Cadaverous-smelling; Putrid; Sour;

Expulsion difficult; Often painless.

Aggravation: Day and night: In scrofulous children: *During dentition:* Before the menses: *During exposure to cold air (pain* and general condition): *After vaccination.*

Amelioration: *From wrapping up warmly* (*pains* and general condition).

During Stool: Chilliness, and nausea in the throat: Colic.

After Stool: Burning and smarting of the anus.

Accompaniments: Obstinacy. Anxiety, excitability, timidity. Rolling of the head from side to side. *Large head, with open fontanelles. Profuse perspiration on the head,* sour-smelling and offensive in the first sleep. Waxy paleness. Pale, earthy-colored face. Loss of appetite; or canine hunger, but on attempting to eat has sudden disgust for food and loses all desire. Much thirst. Aversion to warm, cooked food. Desire for cold things. *Aversion to the mother's milk, and vomiting whenever taking it.* Bitter taste in the morning. Sour eructations. Nausea and vomiting of what is drunk, worse in the morning. Vomiting while drinking, especially if drinking be hasty. Gnawing in the stomach, relieved by drawing up the legs and by eating. *Hard, hot, distended abdomen.* Rumbling of flatulence. Incarceration of flatulence. Discharge of much offensive flatus.

Involuntary urination at night. Suppression of urine.

Restless sleep. Sleepy, but cannot sleep. Feet and legs cold and damp. **Offensive foot-sweat, making the feet sore.**

Emaciation. Want of animal heat, always chilly, even when exercising.

Silic. is one of our most powerful and deep-acting remedies, producing radical changes in the whole constitution, and overcoming fundamental psoric derangements. This renders it often indispensable in infantile diarrhœa and cholera infantum. It most resembles **Calc. c.** The characteristic perspiration on the head differs from that of the latter remedy in being more general over the whole head and forehead. and in the sour, offensive smell. The forehead is also often cold, but becomes warm if lightly covered, which is a very marked symptom of **Silic.** The perspiration under **Merc.** is more oily and sticky.

Mercurius should not be given before or after **Silicea.**

128. STANNUM METALICUM.

Stools: *Green, curdy;* Watery, black; Scanty; Expelled with difficulty.

Aggravation: *In nursing infants:* In children.

During Stool: Colic. Bitter eructations.

Accompaniments: Face pale, sickly looking, flushing easily on exertion. Eyes sunken. Fetid breath. Tongue coated yellow. Canine hunger during the day, with loss of appetite in the evening. Nausea after eating. *The smell of cooking causes vomiting.* Gone feeling in the stomach even after eating. *Colic, relieved by hard pressure, or by laying the abdomen of the child across the knees or against the shoulder of the nurse.* Urine profuse, light-colored or milky. Restlessness. Moaning during sleep. Perspiration, principally on the forehead and nape of the neck, in the morning (after 4 A. M.).

The peculiar colic is the chief indication for **Stannum.**

129. STAPHISAGRIA.

Stools: Yellowish, slimy; Mucous; *Hot;* Excoriating; Bloody; Offensive; *Smelling like rotten eggs;*

Involuntary (when passing flatus).

Aggravation: *After drinking cold water: After eating: In children:* After the least food or drink (colic): After indignation or vexation (colic): After abuse of mercury (general condition).

Before Stool: Cutting pain: Urging.

During Stool: Tenesmus of the bladder and rectum: Discharge of hot flatus.

After Stool: Cutting pain: Itching of the anus.

Accompaniments: Very sensitive to the least impression, either mental or physical. Irritability. Child asks for things and then indignantly pushes them away. Face pale, sunken, sickly; nose pointed; blue rings around the eyes. Mouth and tongue covered with blisters. Salivation. Gums pale, spongy, bleeding when touched. *The teeth, as they appear, turn dark or show dark streaks, and soon crumble. Canine hunger, even when the stomach is full of food.* Absence of thirst. Child cries as soon as it eats. Sensation as if the stomach was hanging down relaxed. Abdomen distended. Hot flatus, smelling like rotten eggs. Cervical glands swollen. Sleepy all day; lies awake all night; body aches all over. Violent yawning and stretching, bringing tears to the eyes. Fetid night-sweats. Bones, especially of fingers, imperfectly developed. Great tenderness and weakness all through the body.

Staph. is too often neglected. It is a valuable remedy for chronic diarrhœa or even dysentery of weak, sickly children, resembling **Cham.** and **Merc.** in many symptoms, but also showing marked and distinctive differences. A humid, fetid eruption is almost always present and furnishes a strong additional indication.

130. STRAMONIUM.

Stools: *Black, fluid; Putrid;* Cadaverous; Painless.

Aggravation: *During typhoid fever:* In childbed.

Amelioration: After profuse perspiration.

Before Stool: Writhing pain in the abdomen.

During Stool: Perspiration.

Accompaniments: Child is very cross and *strikes or bites.* Loquacious delirium, *worse from looking at shining objects; in the dark; when alone. Desire for light and company.* Head drawn to one side; rolling of the head. Spasmodic raising and dropping of the head. Strabismus. Chewing motion of the mouth. Pale face. Diminished appetite. Every kind of food tastes like straw. Violent thirst for large quantities of water. Vomiting of mucus; of green bile. Hard, tympanitic abdomen. Suppression of urine. Constant pulling at the genitals in little boys. Convulsive twitching of arms and legs. Snoring sleep, *with fright on waking;* screaming out during sleep. Fever, with profuse sweat which does not relieve.

The stool of **Stram.** is characteristic when the accompanying symptoms are present.

131. SULPHUR.

Stools: *Watery; Brown, watery* and fecal; *Green, watery, leaving a pale green stain on the diaper; Green, mucous;* Bloody, mucous; Reddish, mucous; Brown, mucous; *White, slimy, mucous;* White, mucous; *Yellow, mucous;* **Bloody in streaks;** *Undigested;* Bilious; *Purulent; Corrosive; Sometimes painless; Changeable; Frothy; Sour; Fetid; Putrid;* Alternating with constipation; Hot; Scanty (bloody or white mucous);

Expulsion sudden and often involuntary.

Aggravation: *In the morning:* **Early in bed**: In the evening and *after midnight:* After taking cold: In damp weather: *After taking milk:* After acids: In children: *During dentition: After suppressed eruptions:* After eating and drinking (colic): *After ale or beer:* From artificial food: *During sleep:* During pregnancy.

Amelioration: By sitting bent and by dry heat (colic).

Before Stool: Sudden and violent urging **(driving one out of bed in the morning without pain)**: *Cutting colic:* Rumbling.

During Stool: Heat: Warm sweat: Rush of blood to the head: Chilliness: Fainting: Nausea: *Tenesmus:* Headache: Soreness in the abdomen: Itching in anus and rectum: Spasmodic constricting pains, extending to the chest, groins, and genitals: Cutting pains, aggravated by pressure or bending backward: *Prolapsus ani:* Drawing knees up to chin: Cramps in the legs: Burning of anus.

After Stool: *Tenesmus:* Burning at the anus: Cold perspiration on the face and feet: *Excoriation about the anus:* Soreness in the whole intestines: Pressure in the rectum: *Prolapsus ani:* **Child falls asleep as soon as the tenesmus ceases.**

Accompaniments: Peevishness or melancholy. Child cross and obstinate. *Open fontanelles. Face pale* or sallow, and covered with cold sweat. Blue rings under the eyes. *Lips very red.* Tongue coated white, with red tip and borders, or brown, parched and cracked. Dry tongue in the morning. Sour, bitter, or putrid taste in the morning. Sweet, nauseating taste. Aphthæ. Ptyalism. Food tastes like straw. *Loss of appetite, with constant thirst. Aversion to meat;* to wine. Desire for ale or brandy. Food tastes too salt. Emptiness at the stomach and canine hunger, causing frequent eating, **particularly about 10 or 11 A. M**. *Voracious appetite. Child grasps everything within reach and thrusts it into its mouth.* Sour eructations, worse after taking milk. *Nausea. Vomiting:* of water; of sour food; of milk; bitter, with cold perspiration on the face. Cutting colic, after a meal, after drinking, better while sitting bent. Pinching colic. Cutting in the abdomen, loins and sacrum, relieved by application of dry heat. Abdomen distended and hard. Passage of fetid flatus. Dysuria. Retention of urine. Urine excoriates the parts. *Excoriation about the anus. Moist excoriation about the genitals.* Labored, heavy breathing. Cramps in the calves and soles, particularly at night. Hands and feet cold, or *palms and soles burning hot.* Ankles weak. *Sleepiness in the daytime, afternoon and after sunset. Sleeping with eyes half open. Wakefulness. Waking often*, with screams. Sudden jerking of the limbs when going to sleep. Child kicks the clothes off at night. *Stupor, with pale face, dropping of lower jaw, eyes half open, cold sweat on the face, suppression of urine and frequent twitching of the muscles.*

Skin harsh, wrinkled; child looks like an old man. **Offensive odor of the body despite frequent washing. Aversion to washing.** Continued dry heat, or coldness and cold sweat. Chilliness about the lower part of the body. Glands swollen, particularly the cervical, axillary and inguinal. Child easily fatigued; sits bent forward; refuses to stand long, but crawls about. *The smell of the stool follows him all around as if he had soiled himself. Excessive prostration and rapid emaciation.*

During Convalescence: Great prostration, with entire loss of appetite and general coldness of the surface.

Sulphur has a very wide range of application, being often required for every kind of loose evacuations by virtue of its similarity, and also, when not distinctively similar, when the appropriate remedies fail to act, or when the improvement which they produce constantly gives way and the patient gets better and worse. The early morning diarrhœa is very characteristic. It is especially useful in dysentery after **Acon.** has removed the acute symptoms, when the tenesmus has ceased, but blood is still discharged.

132. SULPHURIC ACID.

Stools: *Chopped, saffron-yellow, mucous; Stringy; Frothy*, mucous; Watery; *Green, watery;* Black; Undigested; Frequent; Copious;

Offensive, smelling like rotten eggs (watery stool).

Aggravation: *In children:* During dentition: After eating: *After oysters.*

Before stool: Pressing in the anus.

During Stool: Burning in the rectum.

After Stool: Empty, weary, exhausted feeling in the abdomen: Pressing in the anus.

Accompaniments: *Irascibility. Irritability.* Restlessness. Children do everything hurriedly. Profuse flow of tasteless or sweetish saliva. *Aphthæ.* Vesicles on the inside of the cheek. Aversion to the smell of coffee. Desire for fresh fruits. Loss of appetite. Cold sweat on the forehead when eating, even warm food. Cold water chills the stomach unless mixed with some alcoholic liquor. Cough, with belching of wind after coughing.

Sensation of trembling without visible trembling.
Ecchymoses.

Child smells sour, despite the most careful washing.

Great debility and nervous prostration.

The stools and mental symptoms of **Sulph. ac.** are very characteristic, when occurring together, and are mostly met with in children during dentition

133. TABACUM.

Stools: *Yellowish, greenish, slimy;* **Papescent,** fecal; Sudden;

Cholera, without stool, vomiting or thirst.

Aggravation: At night.

During Stool: Colic: *Tenesmus.*

Accompaniments: *Collapse,* anguish and restlessness, death-like pallor, *coldness, fainting, cold perspiration, deathly nausea* without vomiting, or vomiting of water *when moving. Body cold, abdomen hot. Child wants the abdomen uncovered, which relieves the nausea and vomiting.* Great thirst, or thirstlessness. Burning in the stomach. *Coldness in the abdomen.* Hiccough. Vertigo. Oppressed respiration. *Oppression of the heart.*

Icy coldness of the legs from the knees to the toes. Warmth of the body, with icy-cold hands. Cramps in the legs. Hepatic and renal regions sensitive to pressure. *Feeble, irregular pulse.* Spasms or paralysis. *Grinding of the teeth at night.*

Tabac. should not be overlooked in cholera infantum.

134. TARAXACUM.

Stools: Watery; Profuse.

Accompaniments: *Tongue, inside of mouth and fauces covered with a white, slimy coating, peeling off in patches, leaving dark red, sensitive places.* **Mapped tongue.**

Smarting, burning and rawness in the mouth and fauces.

Tough, ropy, sour-tasting saliva.

Throat and larynx feel as if closed.

Frequent hiccough.

Rawness extending from the mouth to the stomach, with burning in the stomach, rising up toward the throat.

Great exhaustion.

Taraxacum can never become a routine remedy for diseases of the bowels; but we may prescribe it with confidence when the above characteristic symptoms of the tongue and buccal cavity are present.

135. TEREBINTHINA.

Stools: *Watery, greenish;* Mucous and watery; *Frequent; Profuse; Fetid.*

Aggravation: In the afternoon and evening: In the morning: During typhoid fever: During nephritis: From living in damp, dark dwellings.

Before Stool: Colicky pains in the abdomen.

After Stool: Violent burning in rectum and anus: *Exhaustion: Fainting*.

Accompaniments: Headache. Vertigo. Flushed face. *Tongue very red, sore and glossy.* **Excessive tympanitis.** Colicky pains in the abdomen. Abdomen tender to pressure. Dull pain and burning in renal region. Pains extending down the ureters. *Burning during urination. Violent strangury. Urine fetid, albuminous, scanty, dark,* **cloudy and smoky. Hæmaturia.** Prostration, with cold, clammy perspiration, and thready, almost imperceptible pulse.

The appearance of the tongue, the meteoristic distension of the abdomen and the urinary symptoms form a group, which unerringly indicates **Terebinth.**

136. THROMBIDIUM.

Stools: *Thin, brown, fecal;* Mucous; *Blood-streaked;* Bloody; Purulent; Mucous and bloody, with hard, fecal lumps;

Frequent; Scanty; *In small, fecal grains, constantly oozing*.

Aggravation: *In the morning: After eating and drinking:* After dinner and supper, but not after breakfast: From fruit: From sugar: In childbed.

Before Stool: *Pain in the left side of the abdomen, with perspiration: Griping pains:* Sore pain in the intestines.

During Stool: *Pain in the abdomen continues: Tenesmus: Chills in the back: Much urging.*

After Stool: *Tenesmus: Prolapsus ani: Burning in the anus:* Great debility: Weakness in the knees: Colic temporarily relieved, but soon returns.

Accompaniments: Fainting on raising up. Loss of appetite. Griping pains in abdomen, aggravated by eating or drinking. Violent colic, causing one to scream with pain. Abdomen very sore.

There has been as yet but little clinical experience with **Thrombidium,** but it has marked and distinctive symptoms, which must render it a valuable addition to the Materia Medica.

It may be distinguished from **Nux vom.** by the immediate concomitants of the evacuations; from **Merc.** by the absence of the sweat and the greenish, bloody stool, so characteristic of the latter remedy; and from **Sulph.** by the aggravation after eating and drinking.

137. THUJA OCCIDENTALIS.

Stools: *Pale yellow, watery;* Oily or greasy; Bloody;

Forcibly expelled; Copious; **Gurgling like water from a bung-hole.**

Aggravation: In the morning: *After breakfast: After coffee:* After fat food: After onions: Periodically returning in the morning, always at the same hour: *After vaccination.*

Before Stool: Rattling of flatulence.
During Stool: Passing of much loud flatus.
After Stool: Debility.

Accompaniments: *Teeth decay at the roots the crown remaining sound.* Much thirst or violent thirst. Drink falls audibly into the stomach. Desire for cold food and drink. *Rapid exhaustion*, causing oppressed and short breathing: irregular and intermittent pulse. *Rapid emaciation*.

It will hardly be easy to make a mistake about **Thuja**. No other remedy has the same combination of symptoms. **Gratiola** resembles it more than any other, but is easily distinguished by the aggravations and accompaniments of **Thuja**. This remedy is applicable to chronic diarrhœa, particularly when traceable to vaccination, or to gonorrhœal infection, and should not be forgotten in cholera morbus, or in cholera infantum. In the latter affections it has a close resemblance to **Laurocerasus**.

138. VALERIANA.

Stools: Thin, watery, with lumps of coagulated milk; Greenish, papescent with blood.

Aggravation: In children: After abuse of Chamomilla, or chamomile tea.

During Stool: Constant pressing and violent screaming.

Accompaniments: Over-excitable, changeable disposition of all the nerves. Jerks, twitches, trembling. Child vomits as soon as it nurses, after the mother has been angry.

139. VERATRUM ALBUM.

Stools: *Greenish, watery, with flakes;* Brownish, watery; *Blackish*, watery; Rice-water; Bloody; *Frequent; Profuse (watery);* Bilious; Mucous; Corrosive; Sometimes painless; Offensive;

Involuntary (while passing flatus).

Aggravation: In hot weather: During or before menstruation: During typhoid fever: *At night:* By moving and drinking (vomiting): After fruit: After indigestible food: From taking cold.

Before Stool: *Severe pinching colic;* Rumbling in the abdomen.

During Stool: *Paleness:* **Cold sweat on the forehead:** *Pinching colic: Nausea: Vomiting: Weakness:* Chilliness and shuddering: Faintness.

After Stool: *Great sinking and empty feeling in the abdomen: Weakness:* Faintness: Great exhaustion.

Accompaniments: Melancholy. Despair. Vertigo with **cold perspiration on the forehead.** Hippocratic countenance. Cold, pale, or bluish face and lips. Sunken eyes. **Contracted pupils.** Lips dry and dark. Tongue cold, or coated white, with red tip and edges, or coated yellow, or dry and cracked. Bitter, sour, or putrid taste. No appetite, or good appetite. *Violent thirst for* *large quantities of very cold water and acid drinks. Desire for fruits; for acids.* Violent nausea with ptyalism. *Violent vomiting: of froth;* of ingesta; of green mucus; of dark green or yellow-green mucus; of sour mucus; of bile. *Vomiting aggravated by drinking, or by the least motion.* Before vomiting, cold hands, becoming hot afterward. *Great weakness after vomiting.* Pressure in the pit of the stomach. Painful retraction of the abdomen during vomiting. Violent colicky pains about the umbilicus, as if the abdomen would be torn open. Abdomen sensitive to pressure. Hoarse, weak voice. Oppressive and spasmodic contraction of the chest. Cold breath. Retention or suppression of urine.

Excessive anguish, arresting the breathing, with desire to sit up or jump out of bed. *Excessive weakness. Fainting.*

Violent cramps of the extremities. Wrinkling of the skin of the hands and fingers.

Skin cold, blue, remaining in folds when pinched.

Veratrum is a remedy of great value, and one very often required, but like all others it demands a careful selection, and is not to be given in every case of cholera morbus or of cholera. The most characteristic symptoms are the same in both cases, only more violent in the latter. The immediate accompaniments of the stool, with the thirst and cravings, distinguish this remedy. **Verat.** is seldom indicated in painless cases.

140. ZINCUM METALLICUM.

Stools: Papescent, enveloped in bright red, foamy blood; Bilious; Thin, pale, bloody; Offensive; Alternating with constipation.

Aggravation: In children: During dentition: In the afternoon, from wine and during rest (general condition).

Before Stool: Colic.

During Stool: Painful tenesmus: Burning at the anus.

After Stool: Tenesmus: Burning at the anus.

Accompaniments: *Child repeats everything said to it.* Face pale, or alternately red and pale. Eyes unnaturally sensitive to light, or fixed and staring. Strabismus. *Forehead cool, base of brain hot.* Grinding of the teeth. Boring of the fingers into the nose, or pulling at the dry lips. Gums bleed on the slightest touch. Tongue white or yellowish-white. Ptyalism. Nausea. Vomiting of water as soon as it reaches the stomach. Hunger, especially about 11 or 12 A.M., with weakness of the legs and trembling. Flatulent distension of the abdomen with rumbling and loud gurgling. Aching; pressure and griping in the sides of the abdomen and umbilical region, with feeling as if the abdominal walls were retracting against the spine. *Urine passed with difficulty, often bloody, and quickly becomes turbid and deposits a yellow sediment.* **Feet constantly in**

motion. Tremulous feeling all over the body. Fainting.

Convulsions: During dentition, with *pale face and no heat, except, perhaps, in the occiput;* ushered in with twitching of single muscles, fidgety feet or loud screams: Gnashing of teeth: Rolling of the eyes: Sharp cries, caused by pain in the head. Automatic motion of hands and head, or of one hand and the head: Coma, the pulse coming in long waves.

Sleep restless with starting, jumping, screaming out, twitching of muscles, and jerking through the whole body during sleep. Wakes frightened, stares, *rolls the head from side to side*.

Zinc. is rarely, if ever, required in the beginning of either diarrhœa or dysentery, but is often useful in later stages, when the cerebral symptoms indicate approaching hydrocephaloid. Deficient nerve power is the great nerve characteristic of the remedy, as shown by the convulsions occurring with pale face and without any increase of temperature. This symptom alone will distinguish **Zinc.** from **Bell.** and other allied remedies.

141. ZINGIBER.

Stools: Brown mucous.

Aggravation: From water containing coal oil: **After drinking impure water**: After taking a chill from a cold, damp wind: After deranging the stomach: In the morning: (After eating melons): After sleep (nausea).

Before Stool: Pinching colic: Difficulty in retaining the stool.

During Stool: Passing of much flatus.

After Stool: Nausea.

Accompaniments: Depression of spirits. Fear that something will happen. Acidity of the stomach. Pains in the stomach. The taste of all food remains in the mouth for hours, particularly of bread or toast. Bad, slimy taste. Frequent eructations. Thirst. Much flatulency, causing rumbling and rolling in the bowels. Nausea. Loss of appetite.

Hæmorrhoidal tumors, hot, and painfully sore, whether sitting or lying. Inflammatory redness, itching, and burning in and around the anus.

If the symptoms of **Zingiber** be further confirmed by clinical observation, it will fill an important place in our therapia. The aggravations are peculiar, particularly the aggravation from drinking impure water.

PART II.
REPERTORY.

PATHOLOGICAL NAMES.

CHOLERA: Acon. *Ars. Camph. Carbo v.* Cicuta, Colch. *Cupr.* Jatr. Phos. Phos. ac. Podo. *Sec.* Sulph. *Tabac.* Thuja, *Verat.*
—, **asphyctica s. sicca**: *Camph. Carbo v. Laur. Tabac.*
—, **infantum**: Acon. Æth. Ant. c. Ant. t. *Ars. Bell. Bis.* Calc. c. Camph. Carbo v. Colch. Coloc. Colost. *Crot. tig.* Elat. Grat. *Ipec.* Iris v. Jatr. Kali bich. Kali brom. Kreos. *Laur.* Phos. Podo. Raph. Sarsap. Sec. *Sil.* Sulph. Tabac. Thuja, Verat.
—, **morbus**: Acon. *Ant. c.* Ant. t. *Ars.* Camph. Colch. Coloc. *Crot. tig. Elat. Grat.* Ipec. Iris v. Jatr. Kali bich. Phos. Phos. ac. *Podo.* Raph. *Sec.* Tabac. Thuja, *Verat.*

DIARRHŒA: Acon. Æscul. Æth. Agar. Aloe, Alum. Amm. m. *Ant. c.* Ant. t. Apis, Arn. *Ars.* Asaf. Asar. E. Asclep. Bapt. Bar. c. Benz. ac. Bol. Bor. Brom. *Bry.* Calc. c. Calc. ph. Canth. Caust. Cham. Chel. *China,*

Cicuta, Cina, Cist. Coccul. Coff. *Coloc.* Con. Cop. *Corn. c. Crot. tig.* Cub. Cyclam. Dig. Diosc. *Dulc.* Ferr. Fluor. ac. Gamb. Gels. Graph. Grat. Hep. Hip. m. *Hyos.* Ign. Iod. Ipec. Iris v. Jabor. Kali bich. Kali c. Kali nit. Kreos. Lach. Laur. Lept. Lil. tig. Lith. c. Magn. c. *Merc. v.* Mez. Mur. ac. Natr. c. Natr. mur. Natr. s. Nicc. Nitr. ac. Nuph. Nux mos. Nux v. Oleand. Op. Ox. ac. Petrol. Phos. Phos. ac. Picric ac. Plant. Plumb. *Podo.* Psor. *Puls.* Raph. Rheum, Rhod. Rhus, Rum. Sabad. Samb. Sang. Scill. Sec. Sep. Staph. Stram. Sulph. Sul. ac. Tabac. Tarax. Tereb. Thromb. Thuja, Verat. Zinc. Zing.

DIARRHŒA, chronic: Æscul. Alum. Amm. m. Ang. Ant. c. Apis, Arn. *Ars.* Asar. E. Bor. Brom. Bry. *Calc. c.* Caust. *China,* Cist. Coloc. Con. Cop. Dulc. *Ferr.* Fluor. ac. Gamb. *Graph. Hep.* Hydroph. *Iod. Kali bich.* Kali c. Kali nit. *Lach.* Lept. Lith. c. *Lyc.* Magn. c. Mez. Natr. c. Natr. mur. *Natr. s.* Nicc. Nitr. ac. *Oleand.* Ox. ac. Petrol. *Phos. Phos. ac.* Podo. Psor. Puls. Raph. Rhod. Rhus, Rum. Scill. Sep. Sil. *Sulph. Thuja,* Verat.

, **infantile:** Acon. *Æth.* Aloe, Amm. m. *Apis, Arg. n. Ars.* Bell. *Benz. ac.* Bis. Bor. *Calc. c. Calc. ph.* Canth. Carbo v. *Cham. China, Cina,* Coff. *Coloc.* Colost. Corn. c. *Crot. tig. Dulc.* Elat. Gamb. *Graph. Hell.* Hep. Ign. *Ipec.* Iris v. Jalap. Kali bich.

Kreos. Lach. *Laur.* Magn. c. *Merc. v.* Natr.
c. Natr. mur. Nicc. Nitr. ac. Nux mos.
Nux v. Oleand. *Paul. Phos.* Phos. ac. *Podo.*
Psor. Puls. Raph. *Rheum*, Sep. Sil. Stann.
Staph. *Sulph.* Sul. ac. Verat. Zinc.

DYSENTERY: *Acon.* Æth. Aloe, Alum. Ant. t.
Apis, Arg. n. Arn. *Ars. Bapt. Bell.* Bol.
Canth. Caps. Carbo v. Caust. China, *Colch.*
Coloc. Cop. Crot. tig. Cub. Cupr. Dulc. Elat.
Gamb. Hep. Hip. m. Hydroph. Ign. Iod.
Ipec. Iris v. *Kali bich. Magn. c. Merc. c.*
Merc. v. Nitr. ac. *Nux v.* Ox. ac. Petrol.
Phos. Psor. Puls. Raph. Rhod. *Rhus*, (Sabad.)
Staph. Sulph. Verat. Zinc.

——-, **periodical in early part of summer,
every year on same month and day:**
Kali bich.

CHARACTER OF THE STOOLS.

Albuminous: Diosc. Natr. m.
Alternating with constipation: Amm. m. Ant.
c. Arg. n. Ars. Bry. Carbol. ac. Chel. Cina,
Coff. Con. Cop. Gamb. Ign. Iod. Kali c.
Lach. Natr. mur. Nux v. Phos. Rhus,
Sulph. Zinc.

—— —— —— **during pregnancy:** Diosc.

—— —— **heat in head:** Bell.

Attack sudden: *Camph.* (Cupr.) *Sec.*
Bilious: Acon. Æth. Agar. Aloe, Ant. t. Ars.
Carbol. ac. *Cham.* China, Cina, Coloc. *Corn.*

c. Cub. Diosc. Dulc. Elat. *Fluor. ac.* Ipec. Lept. Lil. tig. Merc. c. Merc. v. Phos. Podo. *Puls.* Sulph. Verat. Zinc.

Bilious, in albuminuria: Tereb.

Biliary coloring matter, deficiency of: Chel.

Bloody: Acon. Æscul. Æth. Agar. Aloe, Alum. Ant. t. Apis, Arg. n. *Arn.* Ars. Asar. *Bapt.* Bell. Benz. ac. Bol. Bry. Calc. c. *Canth. Caps.* Carbo v. Carbol. ac. Caust. Cham. China, Cina, *Colch. Coloc.* Cop. Crotal. Cub. Cupr. Dulc. Elat. Ferr. Hep. Hip. m. Hydroph. Ign. Iod. Ipec. Iris v. Jalap. *Kali bich.* Kali brom. Kali c. Kali nit. Kreos. Lach. Lept. Lyc. *Merc. c. Merc. v.* Natr. mur. Nitr. ac. Nux mos. *Nux v.* Ox. ac. Natr. s. Paul. Petrol. *Phos.* Plumb. Podo. Psor. Puls. Raph. Rhus, Sabad. Sep. Sil. Staph. Sulph. Thromb. Thuja, Verat. Zinc.

—— and slimy, separated: Mur. ac.

——, black: Alum. *Caps.* Verat.

——, coagulated, copious: Amm. m.

——, ——, dark: Merc. c.

——, decomposed, looking like charred straw: *Lach.*

——, great quantity of: Merc. c.

——, in streaks: Calc. c. Colch. *Sulph.* Thromb. Podo.

Cadaverous: See Smell.

Changeable: Cham. Colch. Dulc. Podo. *Puls.* Sulph.

Coffee grounds, like: Dig.

CHARACTER OF THE STOOLS.

Color, black: Acon. Ant. t. Apis, Ars. Asclep. Bol. *Brom.* Bry. Camph. Caps. Carbo v. China, Cicuta. Cub. Cupr. Hip. m. Iris v. Kali bich. Lept. Merc. v. Natr. mur. Podo. Phos. *Psor. Scill.* Sep. Stann. *Stram.* Sulph. Sul. ac. Tabac. Verat.

———, **bluish**: Phos.

———, **light bluish matter**: Colch.

———, **brown**: Acon. Æscul. Aloe, Ant. t. Apis, Arg. n. *Arn.* Ars. Asaf. Bapt. Bor. Bry. Camph. Canth. Carbo v. Chel. China, Coloc. Ferr. Fluor. ac. Gamb. *Graph.* Grat. Iris v. Kali bich. Kali c. Kreos. Lil. tig. Lyc. Magn. c. Merc. v. Mez. Nux v. Ox. ac. Petrol. Phos. Plant. *Psor. Raph.* Rheum, Rhod. Rum. Sabad. *Scill.* Sec. Sulph. Thromb. Verat. Zinc. Zing.

———, **chalk-like**: Bell. *Calc. c.* Dig. Hep. Lach. Podo.

———, **chocolate-like**: *Ars.* China, *Lach.*

———, **clay-colored**: Hep.

———, **creamy**: Arg. n. Calc. c. *Gels.*

———, **dark**: Arg. n. Bapt. Bol. Carbo v. Hip. m. Nux v. Op. Plumb.

———, **gray**: Aloe. Calc. c. Chel. Cist. *Dig. Kali c.* Merc. v. Natr. mur. Picric ac.

———, **ashy-gray**: Carbo v.

———, **green**: Acon. Æscul. Æth. Agar. Aloe, Alum. Amm. m. Ant. t. Apis, Arg. n. Ars. Asaf. Asclep. Bell. Bor. Brom. Bry. Calc. c. *Calc. ph.* Canth. Cham. China, Cina, Colch.

Coloc. Colost. Corn. c. Crot. tig. Cupr. *Dulc.*
Elat. Gamb. Gels. Grat. *Hep.* Ipec. Iris v.
Kali brom. Kreos. Laur. Lept. Lyc. *Magn. c.*
Merc. c. *Merc. v.* Natr. mur. Natr. s. Nitr.
ac. Nux v. *Paul.* Petrol. Phos. Phos. ac.
Podo. Psor. Puls. Raph. Rheum, Rhus, Sec.
Sep. Stann. Sulph. Sul. ac. Tabac. Tereb.
Verat.

Color, green as grass: Ipec.
——, —— like chopped spinach: Acon.
——, —— like flakes of spinach: Arg. n.
——, —— bright flakes: Paul.
——, greenish: Valer.
——, —— brown, dark: Calc. c.
——, —— mixed with mucous flocculi: Cop.
——, —— turning blue on standing: Phos.
——, —— yellow: Apis.
——, red: Arg. n. Canth. *Cina,* Colch. Graph.
Lyc. Merc. v. *Rhus,* Sil. Sulph.
——, light red: Natr. s.
——, white: Æscul. Amm. m. Ant. c. Apis,
Ars. *Bell. Benz. ac.* Calc. c. Calc. ph. Canth
Caust. Cham. Chel. China, *Cina,* Coccul,
Cop. *Dig. Dulc.* Elat. Graph. *Hell. Hep.*
Ign. Iod. Ipec. Kreos. Lach. Lyc. Merc.
v. *Phos. Phos. ac.* Podo. Puls. Rheum,
Rhus, Sulph.
——, —— jelly-like: Hell.
——, —— grains or particles: Cub. **Phos.**
——, —— masses like tallow: *Magn. c.*
——, whitish: Ang.

CHARACTER OF THE STOOLS.

Color, whitish gray, streaked with blood: Calc. c.

——, **yellow**; Æth. Agar. Aloe, Amm. m. Ang. Ant. c. Ant. t. *Apis*, Arg. n. Arn. Ars. Asaf. Asar. E. Asclep. Bapt. Bar. c. Bell. Bol. Bor. Bov. Brom Calc. c. Canth. Cham. Chel. *China*, Cist. Coccul. Colch. *Coloc.* Colost. *Crot. tig.* Cub. Cyclam. Dig. Diosc. Dulc. Fluor. ac. Gamb. Gels. Grat. *Hep. Hyos.* Ign. Ipec. Iris. v. Jabor. Kali bich. Kali c Lach. Laur. Lept. Lith. c. Lyc. Magn. c. Merc.c. Merc.v. Natr.c. Natr. s. Nicc. Nuph. Nux mos. Oleand. Phos. Phos. ac. Picric ac. Plumb. *Podo*. Puls. Raph. Rheum, Rhus, Samb.Sec.Staph.Sulph.Sul.ac.Tabac. Thuja.

——, —— **bright:** Fluor ac.

——, —— **intense, with green and yellow flakes:** Asclep.

——, —— **like stirred eggs:** Ars.

——, —— **turning green on standing:** Arg. n. Rheum.

——, **yellowish-brown:** Apis, Asar.

——, —— **gray:** Cist.

——, —— **green:** Crot. tig. Grat.

Colorless: Bor.

—— **increasingly, and watery:** Coloc.

Constant discharge: *Apis*, Ox. ac. *Phos*. Sep. *Thromb*.

Copious: Æth. Aloe, Amm. m. Ang. Ant. c. Ant. t. Apis, Arn. Ars. *Asaf. Benz ac*. Bry. Cact. Calc. c. Camph. China, Colch. Colost.

Cop. *Crot. tig*. Cub. Diosc. *Elat*. Gamb. Hydroph. Iod. Iris v. *Jatr*. Kali bich. Kali c. Lept. Lil. tig. Magn. c. Mur. ac. Natr. mur. Nux mos. *Paul*. Phos. Plumb. *Podo*. Raph. Rhus, Rum. Sec. Tarax. Tereb. *Thuja, Verat*.

Corrosive: Acon. Alum. Ant. c. Arg. n. *Ars*. Bapt. Bry. Canth. Cham. China, Colch. Coloc. Colost. Dulc. Ferr. Gamb. *Graph*. Ign. Iris v. Kali c. Kreos. Lach. Lept. *Merc. v.* Natr. mur. Nux v. Phos. Plant. Puls. Rheum, Staph. *Sulph*. Verat.

Epithelial substances, masses of: Arg. n.

Excoriating: See **Corrosive**.

Expulsion difficult: *Alum*. Calc. ph. Gels. Hep. Psor. Sil. Stann.

—— ——, only possible when standing: *Caust*.

—— ——, —— —— —— urinating: Aloe, Alum.

—— forcible, sudden: *Aloe*, Arg. n. *Calc. ph*. Caps. Cicuta, Cist. *Crot. tig*. Cyclam. Dulc. Elat. Ferr. *Gamb. Grat*. Jabor. *Jatr*. Kali bich. Lept. Merc. v. Natr. c. Natr. mur. Natr. s. Nicc. *Phos. Podo*. Raph. Rhod. Sec. Sep. *Sulph*. Tabac. Thuja.

—— ——, like a spout: Crot. tig.

——, gushing: Ferr.

——, sputtering, spattering all over the vessel: Natr. s.

——, squirting out: Elat.

CHARACTER OF THE STOOLS.

Fecal: Acon. Alum. Caust. Chel. Cina, Coff. Dig. Iod. Laur. Mur. ac. Natr. c. Nicc. Ox. ac. Rheum.

——, **black**: Ant. t. Bol. *Brom.* Camph. Cub. Hip. m. Iris v. *Lept.* Sulph. Tabac.

——, —— **and hard, first part, last part white as milk**: Æscul.

——, **brown**: Æscul. Ant. t. *Asaf.* Bor. Bry. Coloc. Fluor. ac. Kali c. Lil. tig. Lyc. Mez. Ox. ac. Petrol. Rheum, Rhod. Rum. Thromb.

——, **dark brown**: Dulc.

——, **light brown**: Æscul.

——, **cream-colored**: Arg. n. Calc. c. *Gels.*

——, **dark**: *Bapt.* Carbo v. Hip. m. Nux v.

——, ——, **first part, last part white**: *Æscul.*

——, **grains, small**: *Thromb.*

——, **gray**: Calc. c. Cist. *Dig. Kali c.* Picric ac.

——, **first part, last part thin and watery**: Bov.

——, **oily-looking**: Bol. *Iod.* Picric ac. Thuja,

——, **papescent**: Æscul. Aloe, Arn. Asaf. Bapt. Bar. c. Bell. Bis. Bry. Calc. ph. Chel. Cyclam. Graph. Hep. Ign. Iris v. Kreos. Lach. Laur. Lept. Petrol. Plant. Podo. Sec. Valer. Zinc.

——, —— **with blood**: Valer.

——, **thin**: Agar. Alum. Arn. *Bapt.* Bol. Bor. Bry. Carbo v. Chel. Cist. Con. Diosc. *Gamb. Hep.* Ign. Iris v. Kali nit. *Lept.* Lyc. (*Nat.*

s.) Nicc. Nux v. Oleand. *Picric ac.* Rheum, Rhod. Rum. Samb Sang. Thromb. Zinc.

Fecal, white: Æscul. *Bell.* Calc. ph. Cop. Dig. Lyc. *Podo.* Rhus.

——, yellow: *Agar. Aloe,* Amm. m. Ant. t. *Apis,* Asaf. Bapt. Bol. Bor. Bov. Calc. c. Chel. Cist. Coccul. Coloc. Cub. Dig. Diosc. Fluor. ac. *Gamb.* Gels. *Hep.* Iris v. Kali c. Lach. Laur. Lith. c. Natr. c. (*Natr. s.*) Oleand. *Phos. ac.* Picric ac. *Podo.* Rhus, Samb.

Fermented: *Arn.* Bor. *Ipec.* Mez. Plant. Rheum, Rhod. Sabad.

Fetid: See **Smell**.

Flakes: Arg. n. Chel. Colch. Cupr. Nitr. ac. Paul. *Verat.*

Flocculi: Cop. Dulc. Sec.

Fluid: See **Liquid**.

Foamy: See **Frothy**.

Frequent: Acet. ac. Acon. Ant. t. Apis, Arg. n. Arn. *Ars.* Bapt. Bell. Bov. Bry. Calc. c. Calc. ph. Canth. *Caps. Carbo v. Cham.* China, Cicuta, Cina, Coccul. Colch. Coloc. Corn. c. Cub *Cupr.* Dulc. *Elat.* Gamb. Grat. Hell. Hyos. Ipec. Iris v. Kali bich. Kali brom. Lach. *Merc. c. Merc. v.* Mez. *Nux v.* Oleand. *Podo.* Psor. Puls. Rhus, Samb. Sec Sep. Tereb. Thromb. Verat.

Frothy: *Arn.* Benz. ac. Bol. *Bor.* Calc. c. Canth. China, *Coloc.* Crot. tig. *Elat. Grat.* Iod. Ipec. *Kali bich. Magn. c.* Merc. v. Natr. s. Op.

CHARACTER OF THE STOOLS. 215

Plant. Podo. Raph. Rheum, Rhus, Sil. *Sulph*. Sul. ac.

Frothy, greenish: Caps.

Glittering grains: Mez.

Glue, like thick, in strips like tape: Carbol. ac.

Gushing: See **Pouring out** and **Shooting out.**

Hot: Aloe, *Calc. ph. Cham.* Cist. Diosc. Merc. v. Phos. Podo. Staph. *Sulph.*

Infrequent, long intervals between: Arn.

Involuntary: Apis, Arg. n. Arn. Ars. Bapt. Bar. c. Bell. Bry. Calc. c. Camph. Carbo v. Carbol. ac. Chel. *China*, Cina, Colch. Con. Cop. Crotal. Cub. Dig. Dulc. Ferr. Gels. Grat. *Hyosc.* Iris v. Kali bich. Kali c. Lach. Laur. Mur. ac. Natr. mur. *Oleand. Op.* Ox. ac. Phos. Phos. ac. Plumb. Psor. Rhus, Sec. Sulph. Sul. ac. Verat. Zinc.

——, **at night in bed:** Carbol. ac.

——, **during sleep:** Arn. Ars. Bell. Bry. China, Con. Hyosc. Mur. ac. Natr. mur. Phos. Phos. ac. Puls. Rhus, Sulph. Verat.

——, **walking, standing, or after eating:** Aloe.

——, **when coughing or sneezing:** *Scill.*

——, **when passing flatus:** Acon. **Aloe,** Bell. Carbo v. Caust. Ign. Kali. c. Mur. ac. Natr. mur. Natr. s. **Oleand.** *Phos. ac.* Podo. Staph. Sulph. Verat.

——, —— —— **urine:** Aloe, Mur. ac. **Natr. s.** Scill. Sulph. Verat.

——, **with every motion:** *Apis.*

CHARACTER OF THE STOOLS.

Jelly-like: See **Mucous gelatinous**.

Liquid: Acet. ac. Æth. Aloe, Ant. t. Bapt. Caust. Chel. Cicuta, Coccul. Coff. Con. Natr. c. Raph. Sabad. Sil. Valer.

———, black: Acon. *Ars.* Carbo v. Carbol. ac. Crotal. *Scill. Stram.*

———, brown: Arg. n. *Graph.* Magn. c. Nux v. Phos. *Psor. Raph. Scill.*

———, dark: Crotal. Op. Scill.

———, green, gradually changing to colorless: Grat.

———, dark green: Crotal.

———, greenish: Æth. Ant. t. Crot. tig. Raph.

———, ——— gray: Æth.

———, otter-colored: Rhus.

———, red, dark: Rhus.

———, reddish-yellow: Lyc.

———, yellowish-white: Nitr. ac.

———, yellow: Æth. Coloc. Crot. tig. Iris v. Lyc. Merc. v. *Natr. s. Nux mos.* Raph. Rhus.

Lumps, gelatinous: Aloe, Chel.

———, like chalk: Bell.

Lumpy: *Ant. c.* Apis, Con. Diosc. Graph. Ipec. Kali bich. Lyc. Thromb.

Masses like tallow: *Magn. c.*

Membranes: *Colch.*

———, false, flakes of: *Nitr. ac.*

———, mucous, shreds of: *Merc. c.*

Milk, like curdled: Gamb.

Mucous: Ang. Ant. c. Ant. t. Arn. Ars. Asaf. Asar. Bell. Bor. Canth. *Caps.* Carbol. ac.

Carbo v. Cham. Chel. China, Cina, Coccul.
Coloc. Corn. c. Cyclam. Dig. Graph. Hell.
Hyosc. Iod. Ipec. Iris v. Kali c. Lept. Merc.
v. Natr. c. Nitr. ac. Nux v. Ox. ac. Petrol.
Phos. Puls. Raph. Rheum, Rhus, Sec. Sep.
Sil. Stann. Staph. Sulph. Thromb. Verat.

Mucous, adhesive: *Caps.*

———, **black**: Ars.

Mucous, bloody: Acon. *Æth. Aloe,* Apis,
Arg. n. Arn. *Ars.* Bapt. Bar. c. Bell. Bol.
Canth. *Caps.* Carbo v. Cham. *Coloc.* Cub. Elat.
Gamb. Hep. Hydroph. Ign. Iod. Iris v.
Lept. Lil. tig. *Merc. c. Merc. v.* Nitr. ac.
Nux v. Ox ac. Petrol. Plumb. Podo. Psor.
Puls. Rhus, Sabad. Sulph. Thromb.

———, **preceded by hard stool**: Bry.

———, **brown**: *Ars.* Bapt. *Carbo v.* Grat. *Nux v.*
Rheum, Zing.

———, **chopped eggs and spinach**: Cham.

———, ———, **white and yellow**: Cham.

———, **colorless**: Hell.

———, **dark**: Arg. n. Bapt. Bol.

———, ———, **brownish-green**: Mur. ac.

———, ———, **like frothy molasses**: *Ipec.*

———, **flaky**: Ferr.

———, **frothy**: Fluor. ac. *Iod.* Podo. Sil. Sul. ac.

———, **gelatinous**: *Aloe,* Apis, Asclep. *Colch.*
(Cub.) Diosc. *Hell.* Kali bich. Mur. ac.
Podo. *Rhus,* Sep.

———, ———, **like frog spawn**: Hell.

———, **granular**: Bell. *Phos.*

Mucous, green: Acon. Æscul. *Æth.* Agar, Amm. m. Ant. t. *Apis*, *Arg. n.* Ars. Bell. Bor. *Bry.* *Calc. ph.* Canth. *Cham.* Chel. Cina, *Coloc.* Corn c. *Dulc.* Elat. Gamb. Hep. *Ipec.* Kreos. *Laur. Magn c. Merc. v.* Nitr. ac. Nux v. *Paul.* Petrol. *Phos.* Phos. ac. Podo. Psor. *Puls.* Rheum, Rhus, Sep. *Sulph.*

——, liquid: *Laur.* Tereb.

——, ——, green: Laur.

——, ——, Carbo v.

——, red: Arg. n. Canth. *Cina*, Colch. Graph. Lyc. Merc. v. *Rhus*, Sil. Sulph.

——, in resinous masses: Asar. E.

——, in shaggy masses: Arg. n. Asar. E. Caps. Lyc.

——, slimy: Acon. Æscul. Æth. Agar. Aloe, Amm. m. Ang. Ant. t. *Apis*, *Arn.* Ars. Bell. Bor. Brom. Calc. c. *Calc. ph.* Caps. Carbo v. Cham. Cicuta, Cina, Coccul. Colch. *Coloc. Corn. c.* Diosc. Dulc. Ferr. Gamb. Hep. Ign. Lach. Magn. c. *Merc. c. Merc. v.* Natr. s. Nux mos. *Nux v.* Petrol. Podo. Rheum, *Rhus*, Sabad. Scill. Sec. Sep. Sil. Staph. Sulph. Tabac.

——, ——, black: Coccul.

——, ——, clear: Puls.

——, ——, grayish-green: Chel.

——, ——, green: Puls.

——, ——, greenish: Podo.

——, ——, like yeast: Ant. t.

——, slimy, pale: Chel.

CHARACTER OF THE STOOLS.

Mucous, slimy, red: Puls.
——, ——, **white:** Cham.
——, ——, **yellow:** Puls.
——, ——, **with ascarides:** Ferr.
——, **stringy:** *Asar. E. Sul. ac.*
——, **tenacious:** *Asar. E. Caps. Crot. tig. Hell.*
——, **thick:** Iod.
——, **thin:** See slimy.
——, **transparent:** Aloe, Colch. Cub. *Rhus.*
——, **watery:** Arg. n. *Iod.* Lept. Tereb.
——, **white:** Ars. Bell. Canth. Caust. **Cham.** Cina, *Coccul.* Colch. Diosc. *Dulc.* Elat. Graph. *Hell.* Ign. *Iod.* Ipec. Ox. ac. **Phos.** Phos. ac. Podo. Puls. Rheum, Sulph.
——, ——, **in masses:** Cop.
——, ——, **like little pieces of popped corn:** Cina.
——, **yellow:** Agar. *Apis, Asar. E.* Bell. *Bor.* Brom. *Cham.* China, *Cub.* Ign. Magn. c. Nicc. Podo. Puls. *Rhus*, Staph. Sulph. Sul. ac.
Offensive: See Smell.
Oily-looking: Bol. Caust. *Iod.* Picric ac. Thuja.
Oozing, constant: *Apis.* Ox. ac. Phos. Sep. Thromb.
Painless: Apis, Arg. n. Arn. Ars. *Bapt. Bis.* (Bol.) *Bor.* Bry. Camph. Cham. **Chel.** China, Coccul. Coff. Colch. Coloc. Crot. **tig.** *Ferr.* Grat. *Hep. Hyos.* Jabor. Kali brom. Kali c. Lyc. Natr. s. Nuph. Phos. ***Phos. ac.*** **Podo.** Psor. Rhus, Rum. *Scill.* Sep. Sil.

Stram. Sulph. Sul. ac. Verat.

Painless, in P. M.: Æscul.

Paint, like dirty white: Phos. ac.

Pappy, Pasty: See **Fecal, papescent.**

Pouring out: Aloe, Crot. tig. *Jatr.* Lept. Merc. v. Natr. c. Phos. *Podo.* Raph. Sulph. *Thuja.*

Profuse: See **Copious.**

Purulent: *Apis, Arn.* Ars. Calc. ph. Canth. Iod. Kali brom. Lach. Lyc. Merc. v. Puls. Sec. Sil. Sulph.

Pus in small points or flakes: Calc. ph.

Putrid: See **Smell.**

Ropy: Kali bich.

Scanty: See **Small.**

Scrapings, like, of intestines: Asclep. Brom. Canth. Carbol. ac. Colch. Coloc. Ferr. Merc. v. Petrol.

——, **like, of meat:** Amm. m.

Sediment, meal-like: Phos. ac. *Podo.*

Shooting out: Cist. *Crot. tig. Grat.* Jabor. Rhod.

Skinny: *Canth. Colch.*

Slimy: See **Mucous, slimy.**

Small: Acon. Aloe, Arg. n. Arn. *Ars.* Asar. E. Bapt. *Bell.* Canth. *Caps.* Cham. Colch. Coloc. Corn. c. Crot. tig. Dulc. *Merc. c. Merc. v.* Mez. *Nux v.* Oleand. Puls. Rhus, Sec. Stann. Sulph. Thromb.

Smell, acid: See **Sour.**

——, **brassy:** Apis.

——, **brown paper burning, like:** Coloc.

Smell, cadaverous: Ant. t. Asclep. *Bis.* *Carbo v. China,* Kreos. *Lach.* Sil. Stram.

——, **carrion, like:** Agar. Apis, Bor. **Lach.** Psor. Rhus.

——, **cheese, rotten, like:** *Bry. Hep.*

——, **coppery:** Iris v.

——, **eggs, rotten, like:** Arg. Nit. Asclep. *Calc. c.* Carbol. ac. **Cham.** *Psor.* Staph. Sul. ac.

——, **fetid:** Acet. ac. Agar. *Arg. n. Arn.* (Bell.) Calc. c. Carbol. ac. Coccul. Grat. Hip. m. Iod. Iris v. Kreos. Lept. Lyc. Nitr. ac. Nuph. Phos. Rhus, Sep. *Sulph.* Tereb.

——, **musty:** *Coloc.*

——, **offensive:** Acet. ac. Aloe, Ant. c. Apis, *Ars.* **Asaf.** Asclep. **Bapt.** *Benz. ac.* Bry. Cicuta, Coff. Colch. *Corn. c.* Crotal. Diosc. Gamb. **Graph.** *Lach.* Lil. tig. Lith. c. Lyc. Mez. Nux v. *Op. Phos. ac.* Plumb. **Psor.** Puls. *Rhus,* Rum. **Scill.** *Sec.* Sul. ac. Verat. Zinc.

——, **putrid:** Acet. ac. *Ars.* **Asaf. Bapt.** Benz. ac. *Bor.* Bry. **Carbo v.** *China, Coloc.* Ipec. Nitr. ac. Nux mos. *Podo.* Sep. Sil. *Stram.*

——, **sour:** Arg. n. Arn. (Bell.) *Calc. c.* Camph. Colch. *Coloc. Colost.* Con. Dulc. Graph. *Hep. Jalap. Magn. c. Merc. v.* Mez. Phos. **Rheum,** Sep. Sil. **Sulph.**

——, **strong, like urine:** Benz. ac.

——, **without (odorless):** Æth. Asar. E. Ferr. Gamb. *Hyosc.* **Paul.** *Rhus.*

Soap-suds, like: *Benz. ac.*

Sour: See Smell.

Strings: Chel.
Tallow masses, like: *Magn. c.*
Tenacious like pitch: Merc. v.
Tomato sauce, like: Apis.
Undigested: Acet. ac. Æth. Aloe, Amm. m. *Ant. c. Arg. n.* Arn. Ars. Asar. Bar. c. Bry. *Calc. c. Calc. ph.* Cham. *China,* Coloc. Con. Crot. tig. Dulc. *Ferr.* Gamb. *Graph. Hep.* Iris v. Jabor. Kreos. Lach. Laur. Lept. Lyc. Magn. c. Nitr. ac. *Nux mos. Oleand. Phos* Phos. ac. *Podo.* Raph. Rhod. Sang. Sec. Stann. *Sulph.* Sul. ac.

—— **food of previous day:** Oleand.

Watery: *Acon.* Æscul. Æth. Agar. Aloe, Amm. m. Ant. c. Ant. t. Apis, *Asaf.* Asar. Asclep. Bapt. Bar. c. Bell. *Bis.* Calc. c. *Calc. ph.* Camph. *Carbo v.* Carbol. ac. Cina, Coccul. Coff. *Colch.* Coloc. *Con.* Cop. Corn. c. Cupr. Dig. Diosc. Ferr. Fluor. ac. Gamb. *Grat.* Hell. Hip. m. Hydroph. Hyos. Ipec. *Iris v. Jalap. Jatr.* Kali brom. Kali nit. Lach. Lept. Merc. v. Mez. Mur. ac. Natr. c. Natr. mur. Nux mos. Oleand. Op. Ox. ac. Phos. *Podo. Puls.* Rhus, Samb. Sang. Sarsap. *Sec. Sulph.* Sul. ac. (Tarax.) *Verat.*

——, **black:** Apis, *Ars.* Asclep. Camph. China, Cupr. Kali bich. Natr. mur. *Psor.* Stann. Verat.

——, ——, **with yellow spots:** Asclep.

——, **bloody:** Aloe, Amm. m. Lach. **Petrol.** Sabad.

CHARACTER OF THE STOOLS.

Watery, bloody, like washings of meat: Canth. *Phos.* Rhus.

———, **brown:** *Ars.* Camph. Canth. Carbo v. Chel. China, Gamb. *Kali bich*. Kreos. Petrol. Plant. Rum. Sulph. Verat.

———, **clay-colored:** Calc. c. Kali bich.

———, **clear (colorless):** Apis, Sec.

———, **containing lumps like frog spawn:** Aloe.

———, **dark:** Plumb.

———, **dirty:** Podo.

———, **flakes, with:** Cupr. Paul. *Verat.*

———, **frothy:** *Elat. Grat. Kali bich. Magn. c.*

———, **green:** Amm. m. Bry. Cham. Colost. Dulc. Gamb. *Grat.* Hep. Ipec. Iris v. Kreos. Laur. Lept. *Magn. c.* Phos. *Podo. Puls.* Sulph. Sul. ac. Tereb. Verat.

———, **green scum, with:** **Magn.** c. *Merc. v.*

———, **rice water:** Camph. Carbol. ac. Chel. Ferr. Verat.

———, **white:** *Benz. ac. Caust. Chel.* Dulc. Kreos. Merc. v. *Phos. Phos. ac.*

———, **yellow:** Æscul. Amm. m. *Apis*, Ars. Bor. *Calc. c.* Canth. Cham. *China*, Colost. Crotal. *Crot. tig*. Cyclam. Dulc. Gamb. *Grat. Hyos.* Ipec. Jabor. Kali bich. *Natr. s.* Nuph. Phos. *Phos. ac.* Plumb. *Rhus, Thuja.*

———, **yellow, containing flakes of mucus:** Chel.

———, **with lumps of coagulated milk:** Valer.

Whey-like: *Iod.*

White, shining particles like kernels of rice: Cub.

CONDITIONS OF THE STOOLS AND OF THE ACCOMPANYING SYMPTOMS.

a. AGGRAVATIONS.

Acids, after: Aloe, *Ant. c.* Apis, Ars. Brom. Bry. Coloc. Lach. *Phos. ac. Sulph.*

——, ——, worse at night when lying: Bry. Lach.

Acute diseases, after: *Carbo v. China, Psor.*

Afternoon, in the: Aloe, Bell. Bor. Calc. c. *China*, Dulc. Laur. Lept. Tereb. Zinc.

——, 4 to 6: Carbo v.

——, 4 to 8: Hell. *Lyc.*

——, 5 to 6: Dig.

——, regularly: Ferr.

Aged persons, in: Ant. c. Carbo v. Coff. Fluor. ac. Gamb. Iod. Op.

—— —— with dark complexions: Nitr. ac.

—— prematurely, with syphilitic mercurial dyscrasia: Fluor. ac.

—— women: Kreos. Natr. s.

Air on the abdomen, from cold: Caust.

——, in cold: Sil.

——, —— —— evening: Natr. s.

——, —— currents of: *Acon.* Caps. Nux v.

Air, in, open: Agar. Amm. m. Coff. Cyclam. Grat.

Ale, after: See **Beer.**

Aloes, after (in lager beer or ale): Mur. ac. *Sulph.*

Alone, when: *Stram.*

Alternate days, on: Alum. China, Fluor. ac. Nitr. ac.

—— ——, **a later hour each time:** Fluor. ac.

Anger, after: Acon. Bry. Cham. Ipec. Nux v.

Ascites, in: Acet. ac.

Autumn, in: Asclep. Bapt. *Colch.* Ipec. Iris v. Merc. c.

Bathing, after: Calc. c. Sarsap.

—— —— **cold:** Ant. c.

Bed, in: Cub.

Beer (ale), after: Chin. Gamb. *Kali bich. Mur. ac.* Sulph.

Bending double: Ant. t. Cocc. *Diosc.*

Breakfast, after: Arg. n. Bor. Ox. ac. *Thuja.*

Burns, after: Ars.

Cabbage, after: (Bry.) Petrol.

Castor oil, after: Bry.

Catarrh or Coryza, after: *Sang.*

——, **with bronchial or intestinal:** Cop.

Chargin, after: Aloe, Bry. Cham. Staph.

Chamomilla, after abuse of: Coff. Valer.

Chest, after pains in the: Sang.

Childbed, in: Asar. E. Cham. Hyos. Phos. *Psor.* Rheum, *Sec. Stram.* Thromb.

Children, in (see also **Dentition**): Æth. Bar. c.

Benz. ac. *Calc. ph. Cham.* Cina, Gamb. Hell. Ipec. Iris v. Kreos. Nux mos. Oleand. Rheum, Sabad. Samb. Sep. Sil. Stann. Staph. Sulph. Sul. ac. Valer. Zinc.

Children, fat: Calc. c.
——, ——, pale: Ipec.
——, tall delicate blonde: Kreos.
——, **fontanelles, with open:** *Apis*, **Calc c.** Calc ph. Ipec. *Merc. v.* Sep. **Sil. Sulph.**

Chilly persons, in: Asar. E.

Chocolate, after: Bor. *Lith. c.*

Cholera, epidemic, during: Camph. Cupr. Phos. Puls.
——, after an attack of: Sec.

Cider, after: Calc. ph.

Climaxis, during: Lach.

Coffee, after: Canth. *Cyclam. Cist.* Fluor. ac. Ign. Ox. ac. Thuja.
——, smell of, after: Sul. ac.

Cold, after taking: *Acon.* Aloe, Ars. Bar. c. *Bell. Bry.* Camph. *Caust. Cham.* China, Coff. Cop. *Dulc.* Elat. Gamb. Graph. Ipec. Natr. c. Nux mos. Nux v. Sulph. Verat. Zing.
——, —— —— in summer: Ant. t.
——, becoming, when: *Coccul.*
—— drinks: Ant. c. *Ars.* Bell. Bry. Carbo v. Coccul. Dulc. Hep. Hip. m. Lept. Natr. c. Nux mos. *Puls.* Rhus, Staph. Sul. ac.
—— food: Ant. c. Coloc. Laur. Lyc. Puls.
—— weather: See **Weather**.

Coolness of evening: Merc. v.

Constipation, after: Alum.
Constitutions, in weakly: Fluor. ac.
Contact, from: Bell. Colch.
Covered, when: Camph. Sec.
Dampness: Puls.
Damp houses, living in: *Natr. s.* Tereb.
—— **places:** Dulc.
—— **weather:** See **Weather**.
Darkness, from: *Stram.*
Day, during the: Amm. m. Ang. Bapt. Canth. Cina, Coccul. Con. Crot. tig. Flucr. ac. Gamb. Hep. Jabor. Kali c. Kali nit. Magn. c. Natr. mur. Natr. s. Nux v. *Petrol.* Scill.
Day and night: Kali c. Merc. c. Sil.
Debauch, after: Ant. c. *Nux v.*
Debility, during: Asar. E.
Dentition, during: Æth. Apis, Arg. n. Ars. Benz. ac. Bor. *Calc. c. Calc. ph. Cham.* China, *Coloc.* Corn. c. Dulc. Gels. Hell. Ign. Ipec. *Kreos.* Magn. c. *Merc. v.* Nux mos Paul. Podo. *Psor. Rheum, Sep. Sil. Sulph.* Sul. ac. Zinc.
Diet, after trivial errors in: Fluor ac.
Dinner, after: Alum. Amm. m. China, Nitr. ac. Nux v. Thromb.
Domestic cares, from: Coff.
Drainage, from bad: Carbol. ac.
Drastic medicines, after: *Nux v.*
Draught, after exposure to: Acon.
Drinking, after: Arg. n. *Ars.* Asaf. Caps. Cina, Coloc. Crot. tig. Cub. Ferr. Fluor. ac. Lach.

Laur. Nux mos. Podo. Sec. Sulph. *Thromb.* Verat.

Drinking, after, cold drinks: See **Cold drinks.**
——, ——, impure water: Zing.
——, ——, on a full stomach: Bry.
——, ——, too much water: Grat.
——, ——, warm drinks: Fluor. ac.

Drinks, alcoholic after: Lach.

Drugging, after: *Nux v.*

Drunkards, in inveterate. China, Lach.

Eating, after (See also **After meals**): Agar. Aloe, Amm. m. Apis, Arg. n. *Ars.* Bor. Bry. Calc. c. Carbo v. Cist. Coloc. Con. Corn. c. **Crot. tig.** Cub. Gamb. Hep. Ign. Iod. Lach. Laur. *Lyc.* Nux mos. Nux v. Phos. Phos. ac. Podo. Raph. Rheum, Rhod. Sec. Staph. Sulph. Sul. ac. *Thromb.* Verat.

Eating, while: Ferr.

Effluvia, noxious: Crotal.

Emaciated persons, in: Calc. c. Iod. Phos.

Emotions, depressing: Coloc. **Gels.** *Phos. ac.*

Eruption, after suppression of: Hep. *Lyc.* Mez. **Sulph.**

Evening, in the: Aloe, Bor. *Bov.* Calc. ph. Canth. Caust. Colch. Cyclam. Dulc. Gels. Ipec. Kali c. Lach. Lept. Lil. tig. Merc. v. Mez. Mur. ac. Nuph. Picric ac. Tereb.

Exanthemata, after suppression of: *Bry.*
——, **during:** Ant. t. Ars. China, Scill.

Exercise, bodily, after: Rhus.

Fat, flabby persons, in: Caps.

Fat, light-haired persons, in: Kali bich.
Fever, during gastric: Arn.
——, —— **hectic:** Asar. E.
——, —— **intermittent:** Coccul. Gels.
——, —— **pernicious:** Camph. Cupr.
——, —— **puerperal:** Carbol. ac.
——, —— **typhoid:** Acet. ac. Alum. Apis, Arg. n. Arn. *Ars. Bapt.* Bell. Bry. Hydroph. *Hyos. Lach. Mur. ac.* Nitr. ac. *Nuph.* Nux mos. *Op.* Phos. ac. *Rhus,* Sec. *Stram.* Tereb. Verat,
Food, artificial, after: Alum. Calc. c. Magn. c. Sulph.
——, **change of, after:** *Nux v.*
——, **farinaceous, after:** Natr. c. Natr. mur. Natr. s.
——, **fat, after:** Ant. c. Carbo v. Cyclam. *Puls.* Thuja.
——, **indigestible, after:** Verat.
——, **rancid, after:** Ars. Carbo v.
——, **rich, after:** Arg. n.
——, **solid, after:** Bapt.
Forenoon, in the: Aloe, Apis, Gamb. Lil. tig. Plant.
Fright and fear, after: Acon. Gels. Ign. *Op.* Verat.
Fruit, after: Acon. Ars. Bor. Bry. Calc. c. Calc. ph. *Carbo v. China, Cist. Coloc.* Crot. tig. Ipec. Lach. Lith. c. Magn. c. Mur. ac. *Puls.* Rheum. Rhod. Thromb. Verat.
——. **sour, after:** Ipec.

Fruit, stewed, after: Bry.
—— **, with milk, after:** Podo.
Game, "high," after: Crotal.
Ginger, after: Nux v.
Glistening objects, looking at: *Stram.*
Gouty subjects: Benz. ac.
Grief: *Coloc. Gels. Ign. Phos. ac.*
Ground, after standing on damp: Elat.
Hair, after cutting: Bell.
Heat of sun or fire, after: Carbo v.
Headache, after: Podo.
Hearing water run: *Hydroph.*
Hereditary in old women: Natr. s.
Hour, at same: Apis.
Hydrocephalus acutus, during: Apis, Bell. Carbol. ac. Hell. Zinc.
Ice-cream, after: *Ars.* Bry. *Carbo v.* Dulc. *Puls.*
Imagination, from exalted: Arg. n.
Indignation: Coloc. Ipec. Staph.
Infants, in nursing: Acon. *Æth.* Bor. Coff. *Jalap.* Kreos. Rheum, Stann.
Injuries, after mechanical: *Arn.*
Jaundice, during: *Dig.* Nux v.
Joy, sudden: *Coff.* Op.
Lead-poisoning, after: Alum.
Light, bright: Bell. Colch.
Liver, affections of: Chel. Corn. c.
Loss of fluids, after: *Carbo v. China,* Phos. ac.
Lying-in, during: See **Childbed.**
Lying: *Diosc.* Ox. ac. Raph.
—— **, left side:** Am. *Phos.*

Lying, on the back: Podo.

——, **on either side**: Bry.

——, **painful side**: Bar. c.

——, **right side**: Phos. ac.

Magnesia, after abuse of: Nux v. Rheum.

Meal, after a (see also **After breakfast**, etc.):
Æth. Alum. Amm. m. *Aloe*, Apis, *Ars.*
Asar. Bor. Brom. *China, Coloc.* Con. Mur.
ac. Natr. c. Rhod.

——, **during**: **Ferr.**

Measles, after: China, Puls.

——, **during**: Scill.

Meat: Ferr. Lept. Sep.

——, **fresh**: *Caust.*

——, **smoked**: Calc. c.

Melons: Zing.

Menses, after: Graph. Lach.

——, **before**: (Apis,) *Bov.* Lach. Sil. Verat.

——, **during**: Amm. m. *Bov.* Caust. Kreos.
Natr. s. Sul. ac. Verat.

Mental exertion, after: Nux v. Picric. ac.
Sabad.

Mercury, after abuse of: Asaf. *Hep.* Lach.
Nitr. ac. Sarsap. Staph.

Milk: Æth. Ars. Bry. *Calc. c.* Con. Kali c. Lyc.
Natr. c. Nicc. Nux mos. Sep. *Sulph.*

——, **boiled**: Natr. c. Nicc. Nitr. ac. Nux mos.
Sep.

—— **and acid fruit**: Podo.

—— —— **water**: Raph.

Morning, in the: Acet. ac. Æth. Alum.

Amm. m. Ang. Ant. c. Apis, Arg. n. **Bor.** *Bov. Bry.* Cist. Cop. Corn. c. Diosc. Ferr. Fluor. ac. Gamb. Hip. m. Hydroph. Iod. Iris v. *Kali bich.* Kali c. Kali nit. Lil. tig. Lith. c. *Lyc.* Merc. v. Mur. ac. *Natr. s.* Nicc. Nitr. ac. Nux mos. Nux v. Oleand. Ox. ac. Petrol. *Phos.* Phos. ac. *Podo. Rum.* Scill. *Sulph.* Thromb. Thuja, Zing.

Morning, after rising: Æth. Agar. Ars. Fluor. ac. Natr. s. Psor.

——, —— —— and moving about: **Bry.** Lept. **Natr. s.**

—— as soon as he rises from bed: Lyc. Sulph.

——, before rising: *Aloe.* Bell. Bov. China, Cicuta, Diosc. Kali bich. Nuph. *Psor. Rum.* **Sulph.**

——, waking one in: Kali bich. Petrol.

——, 6 A. M.: Arg. n.

Mortification with indignation: Ipec.

Motion: Aloe, Apis, Arn. Ars. Bell. **Bry.** Calc. c. *Colch.* Coloc. Crot. tig. Ipec. Merc. c. Mur. ac. Natr. mur. Ox. ac. Rheum, Rum. Tabac. Verat.

——, downward: *Bor.* Cham. (Gels.)

——, from least: Ferr.

Nephritis during: *Tereb.*

Nervous persons, in: Asaf. Asar. E. Ign.

News, bad: **Gels.**

Night, at: Acon. Æth. Aloe, Ang. Ant. c. Ant. t. Arg. n. *Ars.* Asaf. Asclep. Bov. Brom.

Bry. Canth. Caps. Caust. Cham. Chel. *China*,
Cist. Colch. Cub. Dulc. Fluor. ac. Gamb.
Graph. Hip. m. Hydroph. Hyos. Ign. Ipec.
Iris v. Jalap. Kali c. Kreos. Lach. Lith. c.
Merc. v. *Nux mos.* Phos. ac. *Podo. Psor.*
Puls. Rhus. Tabac. Verat.

Night, after midnight: Arg. n. Ars. Asclep.
Cicuta, Fluor. ac. Hip. m. Iris v. Kali c.
Lyc. Merc. cor. *Sulph.*

——, **midnight to noon:** Ars. Cist.

Night-watching: Nux v.

Noise: Colch. Nitr. ac. *Nux v.*

——, **crackling:** Merc. v.

——, **sudden:** Bell. *Bor.*

Noon, at: Jabor.

Nursing, after: Ant. *Crot. tig.*

——, **while:** Coloc.

—— **women:** China.

Onions: Nux v. Thuja.

Opium, after abuse of: *Mur. ac.* Nux v.

Overheating, after: Acon. Aloe, *Ant. c.* Elat.

Oysters: *Brom.* Lyc. *Sul. ac.*

Periodically, at same hour: Apis, Sabad.
Thuja.

——, **an hour later each time:** Fluor. ac.

——, **at same time of year:** Kali bich.

——, **every fourth day:** Sabad.

Persons who take cold easily, in: Nux mos.

Perspiration, suppressed, after: Acon.

Phthisical subjects, in: Acet. ac. Ferr.

Pneumonia, during: Ant. t.

AGGRAVATIONS.

Pork: Ant. c. Cyclam. *Puls.*
Potatoes: *Alum.* Sep.
Pregnancy, during: Ant. c. Ferr. Hell. Lyc. Petrol. Phos. Sep. Sulph.
Pressure: Ant. t. Bell. Cicuta.
—— about the hypochondria: Acon. Arg. n. Caust. Coff. Lach. Laur. Lyc. Merc. v Nux v.
—— at umbilicus: Crot. tig.
Quinine, after abuse of: Ferr. Hep. Lach.
Rest, during: Cyclam. Rhus, *Rhod.* Zinc.
Rheumatism, after: Kali bich.
——, during: Benz. ac. Colch. Rheum.
Riding, when: Coccul. Nux mos. *Petrol.*
Rising from bed: Rhod.
Rising up: *Acon. Bry.* Op. Thromb.
——, after: Coccul.
School girls, in: Calc. ph.
Scrofulous persons, in: Asaf. Bar. c. *Calc. c. Calc. ph.* Caust. Cist. Merc. v. Samb. Sil. Sulph.
Sea-bathing: Sep.
Seashore, at the: Ars. Bry.
Septic, low states: Crotal.
—— matter in food or drink: Crotal.
Shining objects, looking at: *Stram.*
Sitting: Diosc.
Sitting, erect: *Bry.*
Sleep, after: Bell. Lach. Picric ac. Zing.
——, during: Bry. *Sulph.*
Slender persons, in: Phos.

AGGRAVATIONS.

Small-pox, during: Ant. t. Ars. China.
Smell of broth: Colch.
—— —— **eggs**: Colch.
—— —— **fat meat**: Colch.
—— —— **fish**: Colch.
—— —— **food**: Colch.
——, **strong**: Colch. Nux v.
Smoking: Brom.
Sour-kraut: Bry. *Petrol.*
Spirits, after abuse of: Ant. t. Ars. Lach. Nux v.
Spring, in: Iris v. *Lach.* Sarsap.
Standing: Aloe, Coccul. Ign. Lil. tig.
Stomach, after deranging: Ant. c. Petrol. *Puls.* Zing.
Strain, after: *Rhus.*
Sugar, after eating: Ox. ac.
Summer, in (See also **Hot weather**): Acon. Æth. Crotal. Crot. tig. Kali bich. Paul.
Sun, in bright: Agar.
——, **hot**: Camph.
Supper, after: Iris v. Thromb.
Swallowing saliva, when: Colch.
Sweets, after: Arg. n. Calc. c. Crot. tig. *Merc. v.* Thromb.
Syphilitics, in mercurialized: Asaf. Fluor. ac. Benz. ac.
Thinking of the pain, when: *Ox. ac.*
Tobacco: Cham. Ign. Puls.
Thunder-shower, before: Rhod.
——, **during**: Natr. c. Rhod.

Tuberculous patients, in: Carbo v. Oleand.
Uncovering, when: *Nux v.* Rheum.
Urinating, when: Aloe, Alum. Canth. Hyosc.
Vaccination, after: Sil. *Thuja.*
Veal, after eating: *Kali nit.*
Vegetables: Bry. Lept. Natr. c.
Vexation: Calc. ph. *Coloc.* Staph.
——, with indignation: Ipec.
Walking, after: Calc. c.
——, when: *Aloe,* Alum. Merc. v.
Warm food: *Phos.*
Warm room, in: Apis, *Iod.* **Puls.**
Warmth: Puls.
Washed, while being: Podo.
Water, containing coal oil: Zing.
——, hearing run: Hydroph.
Weaning, after: Arg. n.
Weather, change of: *Dulc.* Psor.
——, cold: *Dulc.*
——, colder, when becoming: *Dulc.*
——, damp: Agar. Aloe, Cist. *Natr. s. Rhod.* Rhus, Sulph.
——, ——, cold: Dulc. Merc. v. Nux mos. Rhod. Rhus.
——, dry: Alum.
——, hot: Aloe, Ant. c. Bapt. Bell. *Bry.* Calc. c. Carbo v. China, Colch. Gamb. Iris v. Kali bich. Lach. Magn. c. Merc. v. Mur. ac. Natr. mur. Nux mos. *Podo.* Rheum, Verat.
——, ——, damp: Colch.
——, dry: Asar.

Weather, dry, with cold nights: Acon. *Dulc.*
——, ——, —— —— and damp nights: Asclep.
——, **stormy**: Petrol.
——, **warmer, when becoming**: *Bry.*
Wet, after getting: Acon. Rhus.
—— **feet, after getting**: Nux mos.
Wind, after exposure to cold: *Acon.*
——, —— **cold, damp**: Zing.
——, **with east**: Psor.
Wine, from: *Zinc.*
Winter: Asclep.
Young persons of rapid growth, in: Phos. ac.

b. AMELIORATIONS.

Air, in open: Diosc. Iod. Lyc. Natr. s. **Puls.**
Ale, after: Aloe.
Bending double: Aloe, Arg. n. Bell. Bry. Cast. China, **Coloc.** Cop. Iris v. Lach. Petrol. Podo. Rheum, Rhus, Sulph.
Breakfast, after: Bov. Natr. s. Thromb.
Coffee: Brom. *Coloc.* Corn. c. Phos.
Cold applications: Cyclam. Lyc. *Puls.*
Cool place, in: **Puls.**
Drinks, cold: **Phos.**
——, **hot**: Chel.
Eating, after: Arg. n. *Brom. Chel.* Diosc. Grat. *Hep.* Iod. Jabor. *Lith. c. Lyc.* Natr. c. Nicc. Nitr. ac. *Petrol.* Plant. Sang.
Eructation: *Arg. n.* Grat. Hep. Lyc.
Flatus, by passing: Aloe, Arn. Calc. ph. **Corn.** c. Grat. Hep. Iris v, Kali nit. Mez.

Food, acid: Arg. n.
——, **cold**: Phos.
Heat, dry: Sulph.
——, **external**: Ars.
——, **moist**: *Nux mos.*
Ice-cream: *Phos.*
Loosening the clothing: *Hep. Lyc.*
Lying down: Merc. v. Sabad.
—— **on abdomen**: Aloe, Alum. Calc. *Coloc.* Phos. Rhus.
—— **on back**: Bry.
—— **on side**: Podo.
—— **on right side**: Phos.
Milk, hot: Crot. tig.
Motion: Coloc. Cub. *Diosc.* Nitr. ac. Plant. *Rhus.*
Pressure: Arg. n. Asaf. Bell. Cast. *Coloc.* Diosc. Gamb. Podo.
Rest, during: *Bry.* Ipec. Ox. ac.
Riding, when: *Nitr. ac.*
Rising from bed: Cub. Diosc. Mez.
Rubbing: Diosc. Lyc.
Sitting: Coccul.
Sleep, after: Alum. Crot. tig. *Phos.*
Smoking: Coloc.
Soup, after warm: Acon.
Standing still: Merc.
Stretching: Mez.
Suppressing the stool: Coccul.
Tea, from sipping: Hydroph.
Vomiting, after: Asar. E.

Warm applications: Alum. *Nux mos.* Podo. Rhus.
Warmth of bed: Coloc.
Water, drinking cold: Cupr. **Phos.**
Weather, damp: Asar.
Wine: Chel. Diosc.
Wrapping up warmly: Sil.

ACCOMPANIMENTS OF THE EVACUATIONS.

a. BEFORE STOOL.

Abdomen, aching, sore, in upper part of Bell.
——, **bursting feeling:** Ars.
——, **colic:** Aloe, Alum. Amm. m. Arg. n. Asaf. Asclep. Bapt. Bar. c *Bell.* Bor. Bry. Canth. Caps. *Cham.* China, Colch. **Coloc. Diosc.** Dulc. Gamb. Gels. Graph. Hell. Hip. m. Ipec. Kali c. Kali nit. Lept. Lyc. Mez. Mur. ac. Natr. c. Natr. s. Nitr. ac. Nuph. Ox. ac. Petrol. Phos. Plant. Podo. Puls. *Rheum*, Rhus, Rum. Sep. Tereb. *Verat.* Zinc. Zing.
——, **constrictive feeling:** Ars.
——, **cutting pains:** Acon. Æscul. Æth. Agar. Aloe, Ang. Ant. c. *Ant. t.* Ars. Asar. E. Brom. Bry. Calc ph. Caps. Carbo. v. Cham. Chel. **Coloc.** Con. Crot. tig. Dig. Dulc. Grat. Iris v. *Jalap.* Laur. *Magn. c.* Merc. c. Merc. v. Natr. c. *Nicc.* Nitr. ac. Nux mos.

Nux v. Petrol. Puls. Rhus, Sang. Sarsap. Sec. Staph. *Sulph.*

Abdomen, distress in: Bol.
———, drawing pains: Nitr. ac.
———, distension: Arn.
———, ———, feeling of: Fluor. ac.
———, fermentation in: *Arn. Lyc.*
———, griping: Aloe, Bell. Bry. Fluor. ac. Psor.
———, ———, with backache: Cub.
———, heat: Bell.
———, left side, pain in: *Thromb.*
———, pinching pains: Æth. Agar. Bell. Bry. Calc. ph. Canth. Cina, Colch. Cyclam. Fluor. ac. *Gamb. Kali c. Magn. c.* Merc. v. Natr. s. Nicc. Petrol. Sabad. *Verat.* Zing.
———, rumbling, rattling of flatus: Æscul. Agar. Aloe, Ant. t. Apis, Ars. Asclep. Bis. Brom. Carbo v. Chel. Colch. Grat. Ign. Iris v. Kali c. Lach. Lept. Mur. ac. Natr. c. Natr. mur. *Natr. s.* Oleand. Phos. *Puls.* Sabad. Sec. Sulph. Thuja, Verat.
———, ——— in right and lower portion of: Aloe.
———, severe pain as though being stepped on, relieved in no position: Iod.
———, ——— ——— in lower part of: Fluor. ac.
———, tearing pains: Dig. Rhus.
———, twisting pains: Aloe, Ars. Caust. Ox. ac. Stram.
———, upper, pain in: Aloe.
———, violent pain: Asclep. Elat. Gamb.
Anguish: Acon. Merc. v.

Anus, burning pains: Fluor. ac. Oleand.
——, constriction of: Plumb.
——, pressing: Arn. Bell. Sul. ac.
——, prolapsus: Podo.
——, soreness: Bar. c.
——, stitches in: Gamb.
Anxiety: Ars. Cham. Crot. tig. Merc. v.
Back, coldness in: Ars.
——, pains in: Bapt. Cicuta, *Nux v.* Puls.
Chest, feeling of hot water pouring from, into abdomen: Sang.
Chilliness: Ars. Bapt. Bar. c. Benz. ac. Dig. *Merc. v.* Mez. Phos.
——, mingled with heat: Merc. v.
Difficulty of retaining stool: *Aloe,* Cicuta, *Sulph.*
Fainting: Ars. *Dig.*
Flatus, passing: Æscul. Aloe, Apis, Arg. n. Asaf. Gels. Mez. Plant. Sabad.
——, ——, desire for, but knows not whether wind or feces escape: Natr. m.
——, —— hot: Aloe, Coccul.
Genitals, pressing toward: Bell.
Groins, pain in: Natr. s.
——, pressing in: *Thromb.*
Head, rush of blood to: Aloe.
Headache: Ox. ac.
Heat: Crot. tig. Magn. c. Merc. v. Phos.
Ill humor: Bor. *Calc. c.*
Intestines, burning: Aloe.
——, gurgling, as of fluid running: Podo.

Intestines, prickling: Aloe.
——, sore pain: Thromb.
Lassitude: Rhus.
Limbs, pain in: Bapt.
Mucus, white, discharge of: Kali c.
Nausea: Acon. Ang. Ant. t. Bry. Calc. c. Chel. Dulc. Grat. Hell. Ipec. *Merc. v. Rhus*, Rum. *Sep*.
Navel, burning about: Ars.
——, cutting about, excessive: Gamb.
——, pain about: *Aloe, Amm. m.* Caps. Fluor. ac. Grat. Nux v. Ox. ac.
——, pain about, relieved by bending double: Aloe.
——, pinching about: Bry.
Pain, rarely: Ferr.
Peevishness: Bor.
Pelvis, fulness and weight in: Aloe.
Perspiration: Acon. Bel. Dulc. Merc. v. *Thromb*.
Plug, feeling of, between symphysis pubis and coccyx: Aloe.
Ptyalism: Fluor. ac.
Rectum, burning in: Aloe, Coccul.
——, chilliness in: Lyc.
——, constriction in: Bell.
——, creeping in: Mez.
——, cutting in: Aloe.
——, dragging down and pressure in: Lil. tig.
——, feels full of fluid: Aloe.
——, feeling of insecurity in: **Aloe**.

Rectum, sensation in, as if it would protrude: Ang.

———, **stitches in:** Asar. E.

———, **sudden, darting pains in:** Apis.

Sacrum, drawing pains in: Carbo v. Diosc. Natr. c.

———, **continuous pains:** Aloe.

Screaming, violent: Ars.

Tenesmus: Bol. *Merc. c. Merc. v.*

Thirst: Ars.

Trembling: Merc. v.

Urging: *Aloe*, Amm. m. Apis, Arn. Asaf. Bor. Bov. Canth. *Cist.* Coccul. Colch. *Coloc.* Corn. c. Gamb. Ign. *Kali bich.* Kali nit. Lach. Lept. *Merc. c. Merc. v.* Mur. ac. Natr. c. Nicc. *Nux v.* Phos. Plumb. *Rheum*, Rhus, Sabad. Samb. Sang. Staph. *Sulph.*

———, **constant:** Bry. Carbol. ac. Elat.

———, ——— **with colicky pain:** Gamb.

———, **ineffectual:** Bar. c. Benz. ac. Bry. Carbol. Nux v.

———, **irresistible:** *Cist.*

———, **sudden:** Æscul. Arg. n. Bar. c. Cicuta, *Cist.* Hip. m. Kali c. *Lil. tig.* Merc. v. Petrol. Phos. Podo. **Sulph.**

——— **to urinate:** Rheum.

Vomiting: Ars. Dig. Ipec.

b. During Stool.

Abdomen, bearing down in: Arg. n.

———, **bruised pain in:** Arg. n. Arn.

Abdomen, colic: Agar. Alum. Ant. t. Arg. n. Ars. Asaf. Asclep. Bapt. Bis. Canth. Caps. Carbol. ac. *Cham. Coloch.* Colost. Cop. Corn. c. Crotal. Crot. tig. Cyclam. Dulc. Hip. m. Ipec. Kali c. Lyc. Magn. c. Mez. Mur. ac. Nitr. ac. Nux v. Ox. ac. Petrol. Podo. Rheum, Rhus, Sil. Stan. Tabac.

——, **constricting pains in:** Arg. n. Sulph.

——, **contraction in painful:** Æth.

——, **cramping pains in:** Iris v.

——, **cutting pains:** Acon. Agar. *Aloe,* Arn. Ars. Asar. e. Bov. Caps. Chel. Coloch. *Coloc.* Crot. tig. Cub. Dig. Elat. Gamb. Iod. Iris v. Jalap. Kali nit. Merc. c. Merc. v. Rhus, Sec.

——, **drawing in of:** Agar. *Plum.* Podo.

——, **feeling of a stream of fire through:** Asclep.

——, **fermentation:** Agar. Bry.

——, **gnawing pains:** Kali bich.

——, **griping pains:** Aloe, Apis, Cub. Plant. *Thromb.*

——, —— —— **with backache:** Cub.

——, **heat of:** Alum.

——, **left side, pain in:** *Thromb.*

——, **pains causing dyspnœa:** Coccul.

——, —— **extending down thighs:** Coloc.

——, —— **pinching:** Agar. Apis, Canth. Merc. v. *Verat.*

——, **pressure in:** Arn. Brom.

——, **rumbling:** Arn. Chel. Corn. c. Cub.

Abdomen, sensation as if bowels would protrude: Kali brom.

——, **soreness in:** Arg. n. Sulph.

——, **squeezing pain in:** Apis.

——, **tearing pains:** Aloe, Cop. Dig.

——, **tenderness of:** Alum.

——, **twisting pains:** Bov.

Anguish: Merc. v.

Anus, biting at: Caps. Lyc.

——, **burning or heat:** *Aloe*, Ant. t. **Ars.** Bar. c. Bel. Bry. *Canth.* Carbo v. Cham. Coloc. Corn c. Cyclam. Ferr. Gamb. Hip. m. **Iris v.** Lach. Lyc. Mur. ac. Natr. c. Natr. s. Nicc. Op. Picric ac. Zinc.

——, **constricted, painful about fallen rectum:** Mez.

——, **cutting in:** Agar. Ars.

Anus, itching at: Sulph.

——, **pain:** Canth. China, Colch. Mur. ac. *Ox. ac. Plumb.*

——, ——, **jerking upward through the rectum:** Sep.

——, **prolapsus:** Asar. Bry. Colch. *Ign.* Mur. ac. *Podo.* Sep. Sulph.

——, **rawness and soreness:** Apis.

——, **smarting:** Agar. China, Kali c. *Mur. ac.* Picric ac.

——, **soreness in:** Grat.

——, ——, **burning in:** Agar.

——, **stinging at:** Caps.

——, **unpleasant sensation:** Æscul.

Anxiety: Cham. Merc. v.

Ascarides, discharge of: Asclep. Calc. c.

Back, chill in: *Thromb.*

——, **pain**: Æscul. Amm. m. Apis, Caps. *Nux v.* Puls.

——, ——, **bruised, in**: Arn.

——, ——, **in small of**: Colch.

Bladder, pressure on: Bell.

——, **tenesmus of**: *Canth. Lil. tig.* **Merc. c.** Staph.

Blood, dropping of: Alum.

——, **discharge of**: Amm. m.

Borborygmus: Colch.

Chill, shaking: Puls. Verat.

Chilliness: Aloe, Ars. Bry. Colch. Cop. Ipec. Lyc. *Merc. v.* Rheum, Sec. Sil. Sulph. Thromb. Verat.

——, **mingled with heat**: Merc. v.

Cramps in the legs: Sulph.

Drawing knees up to chin: Sulph.

Drowsiness: Bry. Corn. c.

Eructations: Cham. Dulc. *Merc. v.* Stann.

Exhaustion: Crotal. Sec. *Verat.*

Extremities, pain in: Amm. m.

Face, congestion to: Aloe.

Fainting: Aloe, Crotal. Sars. Sulph.

Faintness: Bov. Cóccul. Colch. Crot. tig. Dulc. Plant. Verat.

Flatus, passing of: Acon. *Agar. Aloe,* Apis, Arg. n. Asaf. Bis. Brom. China, Coccul. Coloc. Corn. c. Gamb. Hip. m. *Ign.* Laur.

Mur. ac. *Natr. s.* Podo. Samb. Sang. Sarsap. Staph. Zing.

Flatus, passing of, fetid: Æscul. Bry. *Calc. ph.* Carbo v. Diosc. Iris v. *Phos. ac.*

——, —— **noisy:** *Arg. n.* Thuja.

Headache: Apis, Cub. Ox. ac. Sulph.

Head, congestion to: Aloe, Rhus, Sulph.

——, **dulness of:** Corn. c.

——, **heat in:** Ox. ac.

——, **fore-, cold sweat on:** *Verat.*

——, ——, **warm sweat on:** *Merc. v.*

——, ——, **tensive pain:** Coloc.

Heat: Aloe, Dulc. Merc. v. Sulph.

Hæmorrhoids: *Brom.* Fluor. ac. Phos.

——, **distension of:** Ang.

Hunger: *Aloe.*

Intestines, bruised pain in: *Apis.*

Liver, distress in region of: Aloe.

Loins, pains in, to legs: Agar.

Nausea: Agar. Ant. t. Apis, Arg. n. Ars. Bell. Carbol. ac. Cham. Chel. Colch. Coloc. Cop. Corn. c. Crotal. Crot. tig. Grat. Hell. *Ipec. Merc. v.* Nitr. ac. Sil. Sulph. *Verat.*

Navel, burning about: Ars.

——, **pain about:** Fluor. ac. *Kali bich.* Ox. ac.

——, ——, **griping from, to rectum:** Coloc.

Paleness: Calc. c. Ipec. *Verat.*

Palpitation: Ant. t. Cyclam. Nitr. ac. Sulph.

Perspiration: Acon. Agar. Bell. Cham. Coccul. Corn. c. Crot. tig. Dulc. Jatr. Merc. v. Stram. Thromb.

Perspiration, cold: Merc. v. *Verat.*
——, ——, **on limbs:** Gamb.
——, **warm:** Sulph.
Prostration: See **Weakness.**
Rectum, burning in: Aloe, Alum. Amm. m. Ang. *Ars.* Bar. c. Bor. Caps. Coccul. Con. Corn. c. Cub. Diosc. Graph. Sul. ac.
——, **contracted feeling in:** Ars.
——, **cutting in:** Agar.
——, **pain:** Ant. c.
——, ——, **burning:** Grat.
——, ——, **cramping:** Arg. n.
——, **pressure in:** Lyc.
——, **protrusion of:** Ant. c. Canth. Crot. tig. Dulc. Ferr. Fluor. ac. *Ign.* Mez. Plant.
——, **rawness in:** Caps.
——, **scraping in:** Crot. tig.
——, **smarting:** Phos.
——, **stinging:** Nicc.
——, **tearing pains:** Calc. c.
——, **throbbing in:** *Caps.*
——, **unpleasant sensation in:** Æscul.
Sacrum, burning in: Caps.
——, **pain in:** *Æscul.* Podo.
Screaming: Colch. *Merc. v.* Rheum, Valer.
Sexual excitement: Natr. c. Natr. s.
Shuddering: Bell.
Stomach, burning in: Hip. m.
——, **drawing in of:** Agar.
——, **pain in:** Bry.
——, ——, **pressing in:** Bell.

Stomach, pressing in: Brom.
Strangury: Caps.
Taste, nauseous: Crot. tig.
Tenesmus: *Acon.* Æscul. *Æth. Aloe,* Alum. Amm. m. Ang. Ant. t. Apis, Arg. n. Arn. *Ars.* Asclep. Bapt. *Bell.* Caps. Carbol. ac. Caust. *Colch.* Coloc. Con. Cop. Corn. c. Crot. tig. Diosc. Ferr. Fluor. ac. Graph. Grat. Hell. Hep. Hip. m. Hydroph. Ipec. Iris v. *Kali bich.* Kali nit. Lach. Laur. Lil. tig. *Magn. c.* **Merc. c. Merc. v.** Natr. c. Natr. s. Nicc. Nitr. ac. *Nux v.* Op. Petrol. Phyt. Plant. Plumb. Podo. *Rhus,* Sulph. *Tabac. Thromb.* Zinc.

———, **of bladder and rectum:** Arn. Lil. tig. *Staph.*

Thighs, tearing pains down: Rhus.
Thirst: Bry. Cham. China, Dulc. Podo.
Urethra, burning in: Coloc.
Urging: Aloe, Apis, Arg. n. Arn. Benz. ac. *Canth.* Cyclam. Gamb. Hell. *Kali bich.* Magn. c. *Merc. c. Merc. v.* Mez. Nicc. Nux mos. Ox. ac. Rhus, Thromb.

———, **constant:** Valer.
———, **directly on wiping:** Calc. ph.
———, **to urinate:** Aloe, *Alum.* Cicuta, Cub.

Urination: Bell.
———, **involuntary:** *Alum.* Kali brom.
———, **painful, frequent:** Apis.
———, **profuse:** Bry.

Uterus, bearing down pain in: Bell.

Vertigo: Caust. Cham. Stram. Zinc.
Vomiting: Apis, Ars. Bry. Coccul. Colch. Cop.
 Crot tig. Dulc. Elat. **Ipec.** Merc. v. *Verat.*
——— **and urination simultaneously:** Crotal.
Weakness: Æscul. Colch. Plant.
Weariness: Bor.
Worms, discharge of round: Cina.

c. After Stool.

Abdomen, burning in: Bol. Kali bich. Sabad.
———, **colic:** Amm. m. Asclep. Corn. c. Diosc. Nicc. Puls. Rheum.
———, **cutting·** Ars. **Coloc.** Kali nit. *Lept.* Merc. c. Merc. v. Podo. Rheum, Staph.
———, **distension of:** Agar.
———, **empty feeling:** Sul. ac. *Verat.*
———, **heaviness in:** Agar.
———, **pain in:** Æscul. Fluor. ac.
———, ———, **severe in lower:** Gamb.
———, **pinching:** Cyclam. Kali c. Merc. v.
———, **pressing in:** Grat.
———, **rumbling:** Bol. Chel.
———, ———, **and gurgling in left side of:** Crot. tig.
———, **sinking:** *Verat.*
———, **soreness in:** Sulph.
———, **weakness in:** Diosc. Lept. *Phos.* Podo. Sul. ac.
Air, aversion of cold, open: Mez.
Anguish: Acon.

Anus, biting in: Agar. *Canth*.
—, **burning in**: Agar. *Aloe*, Ant. t. **Ars**. Bar. c. Bov *Canth*. Caps. Carbo v. Cicuta, Coloc. Corn. c. Crot. tig. Dulc. Ferr. Gamb. Grat. Hell. **Iris v.** *Kali c.* Kali nit. Lach. Laur. Lil. tig. Magn. c. *Merc. v.* Natr. s. Nitr. ac. Nuph. Nux v. Oleand. Phos. Picric ac. Sil. Sulph. Tereb. *Thromb.* Zinc.
—, —, **as if grains of barley were sticking there**: Nicc.
—, **constriction in**: *Ign.* Lach.
—, **itching**: Aloe, Bov. Carbo v. *Merc. v.* Nicc. Staph.
—, **pains**: Asclep. Colch. Coloc.
—, **pressing**: Sul. ac.
—, **pricking**: Iris v.
—, **prolapsus**: Ars. Asar. E. Ign. Hip. m. Merc. *Podo.* Sep. Sulph. *Thromb.*
—, **pulsation**: Hip. m.
—, **smarting**: Agar. *Canth.* Gamb. Graph. Hell. Lil. tig. Nuph. Nux mos. Picric ac. Puls. Sil. Sulph.
—, **soreness**: Alum. Ant. c. Apis, Cham. Gamb. Graph. *Merc. v.* **Mur.** ac. Nitr. ac. Nux mos. Podo. Sulph.
—, **sore pustules near**: Amm. m.
—, **stinging**: *Canth.* Kali nit. Nicc.
—, **throbbing as from little hammers in**: Lach.
—, **weight**: *Aloe.*
Anxiety: Nitr. ac.

Back, flashes of heat up: Podo.
———, **pain in**: Caps. Hydroph. Merc. v.
———, **small of, chilliness**: *Puls.*
———, ——— ———, **pain relieved**: Ox. ac.
———, **throbbing**: Alum.
Calves, cramps in: Ox. ac.
——— ——— **in right**: Thromb.
Cheerfulness: Bor. Natr. s.
Chest, pains in: Agar.
Chilliness: *Canth.* Grat. Mez.
Coccyx, pains, wrenching in: Grat.
Coldness of body: Crot. tig.
Discharge of white viscid bloody mucus: Asar.
Drowsiness: Æth. Bry. Colch. *Nux mos.*
Dulness and forgetfulness: Cyclam.
Eructations: Ars. Merc. v.
———, **tasting of the ingesta**: Æscul.
Exhaustion: Æth. Aloe, Apis, Ars. Bis. China, *Colch.* Coloc. Crotal. Crot. tig. Graph. Lil. tig. Merc. v. Nitr. ac. Phos. Picric ac. Podo. *Sec. Sep. Tereb. Verat.*
Extremities, lower, pains in: Rhus.
Face, shivering over: Ang.
———, **sunken and altered**: Crot. tig.
Fainting: *Aloe*, Coccul. Crot. tig. Phos. Tereb.
Faintness: Apis, Canth. *Con.* Dig. Lept. Merc. v. *Sarsap.* Verat.
Hæmorrhoids: *Aloe, Brom.* Calc. ph. Diosc. Graph.
———, **blue**: Lach. *Mur. ac.*

AFTER STOOL.

Headache worse: Agar.
Heat: Bry.
Hiccough: Merc. v.
Hunger, canine: Lept. *Petrol*.
Hypogastrium, griping in: Agar.
Irritation, ill humor: Nitr. ac.
Knees, weakness in: Thromb.
Lie down, obliged to: Arn.
Liver, burning pain and distress in: Bol.
Loins, pains in, to legs: Agar.
Nausea: Acon. *Caust*. Hydroph. Crot. tig. Kali bich. Ox. ac. Zing.
——, **with retching**: Kali bich.
Navel, heaviness around: Agar.
——, **pain about**: Aloe, *Lept*.
——, **pressing in**: Crot. tig.
Nervous erethism, great: Ign.
Palpitation of the heart: Ars. Con.
Perspiration: Acon. Ars.
—— **on forehead**: Crot. tig.
——, **cold**: Aloe.
——, ——, **on face**: Sulph.
——, ——, **on feet**: Sulph.
——, ——, **on forehead**: Merc. v. **Verat.**
——, **warm, becomes cold and sticky**: *Merc. v.*
Prostration: See **Weakness**.
Rectum, burning in: Amm. m. *Ars*. Corn. c. Lil. tig. Sabad. *Tereb*.
——, **constriction in**: Merc. v.
——, **heat in**: Apis.
——, **oozing from**: Carbo v.

Rectum, pain: Asclep. Hydroph. Natr. c.
——, ——, burning in: Grat.
——, ——, cramping in: Ferr.
——, —— , violent, cutting, long-lasting: *Nitr. ac.*
——, pressure in: Sulph.
——, prolapsus: Ant. c. Cicuta, Coccul. Crot. tig. Ign. Iris v. *Merc. v.* Mez.
——, ——, becomes constricted:
——, sensation as if plugged: Apis.
——, smarting in: Asclep.
——, stitches in: Cham.
——, straining in: Agar.
——, throbbing in: Apis.
——, tingling in: China.
——, weak feeling in: Lept.
——, weight in: Rhus.
Relief of colic, tenesmus and urging: Acon. Æscul. Aloe, Alum. Ant. t. Arn. Ars. Asaf. Bapt. Bry. Calc. ph. Canth. Cham. Colch. *Coloch.* Corn. c. Dulc. Gamb. Hell. Natr. s. Nuph. *Nux v. Rhus.*
Relief, except of dull, heavy pain in abdomen and back: Cub.
——, of head symptom: Corn. c.
——, of pain: Arg. n.
——. —— —— in abdomen: Arn.
Sacrum, burning along: Coloc.
——, pains from, down legs; Rhus.
Shuddering: Canth.
—— after drinking: *Caps.*

Sleep as soon as tenesmus ceases: *Colch.* Sulph.

Solar plexus, distress in: Bol.

Stomach, burning pain and distress in: Bol.
——, pressure in: Crot. tig.

Stool, feeling as though more would pass: Aloe, Nux mos. Nux v.

Sweat: See **Perspiration.**

Tenesmus: Amm. m. Ant. t. Asar. Bapt. *Bell.* Bol. Bov. *Canth. Caps.* Coccul. *Colch.* Cub. Dulc. Fluor. ac. Hydroph. *Ign.* Ipec. *Kali bich.* Kali nit. Lach. Lil. tig. *Magn. c.* **Merc. c. Merc. v.** Nicc. Phos. Plumb. *Rheum,* Rhus, *Sulph. Thromb.* Zinc.

—— extending to perineum and urethra: Mez.
—— —— up along the sacrum: Puls.
——, with passage of blood: Apis.

Thirst: *Caps.* Dulc. Ox. ac. Thromb.

Throat, dryness of: Ox. ac.

Urging, unsatisfied: *Æth.* Aloe, Ang. Bar. c. Cicuta, Crot. tig. Cyclam. Dig. Lach. Lyc. *Merc. c. Merc. v.* Nicc. *Nux v.* Petrol. Rheum, Samb.

Urination, involuntary: Alum.

Vertigo: Caust. Crot. tig. Petrol.

Vomiting: Arg. n.

Water-brash: *Caust.*

Weakness: Ars. Bov. Calc. c. Carbo v. *Con.* Dulc. Ipec. Mez. Natr. mur. Petrol. Podo. Sep. *Thromb.* Thuja, *Verat.*

GENERAL ACCOMPANIMENTS.

1. Mind and Mood.

Agitated, constantly: Carbol. ac.
Agitation, nervous: Valer.
Anger: Aloe, Ars. Bar. c.
—— when consoled: *Natr. mur.*
Anguish: *Ars. Camph.* Raph. Sil. Tabac. Verat.
Anxiety: *Acon.* Amm. m. Asaf. Calc. c. Canth. *Carbo v.* Cicuta, Fluor. ac. Kali brom. Lil. tig. Magn. c. Merc. v. Psor. Sec.
—— concerning the illness: Nitr. ac. Psor.
—— when lifted from the cradle, expression of: *Calc. c.*
Apathy: Bor. Camph. Colost. *Jatr.* Op. **Phos. ac.**
Aversion to being disturbed: *Bry.* Gels.
—— —— —— looked at: *Ant. c. Ant. t.* Arg. n.
—— —— —— touched: *Ant. c. Ant. t.* Arg. n.
—— —— downward motion: Bor. Cham. Gels.
—— —— light: Bry. Camph.
—— —— mental or bodily exertion: Corn. c. Hep. Rhod.
—— —— noise: Bry. Kali c. Nitr. ac. *Nux v.*
—— —— open air: Aloe, *Nux v.* Petrol.
—— —— sound of scratching on cloth: Asar. E.
—— —— washing: *Sulph.*
—— —— —— cold: *Ant c.*
Carphologia: Hyos. Op.

Changeable mood: Alum. Valer.
Clumsiness: Asaf.
Cowardice: Bar. c.
Cries, piercing: Apis, Carbol. ac.
Crying: Æth. Alum. Ars. Bell. *Bor.* Calc. c. Caust. *Cham.* Cina, Psor. Puls.
Delirium: Bapt. Bell. Bry. Canth. Carbol. ac. *Hyos.* Mur. ac. Op. Phos. ac. Rhus, *Stram.*
—— alternating with colic: *Plumb.*
——, merry, loquacious: Agar.
Depression, sadness, despondency, melancholy: Æscul. Alum. Asclep. Bol. Calc. ph. Chel. Crotal. Cyclam. Gamb. Hep. *Ign.* Iris v. Kali bich. Lil. tig. Lyc. Natr. c. *Natr. mur.* Nitr. ac. Plant. **Puls.** Sulph. Verat. Zing.
Desire for company: Bis. *Stram.*
—— —— light: *Stram.*
—— —— many things, rejected when offered: Ang. Cham. *Cina*, Staph.
—— —— open air: Puls.
—— to be carried: *Cham.*
—— —— —— covered: Hepar, **Nux** v.
—— —— —— naked: *Hyos.*
—— —— —— quiet: *Bry.* Gels.
—— to draw a deep breath: *Ign.* Natr. s.
—— —— have abdomen uncovered: *Tabac.*
Dulness, almost idiocy: Agar.
Distrustful mood: Ant. c.
Excitability: Agar. *Coff.* Gels. Lil. tig. Phos. Psor. Samb. Sil. Valer.

Exhilaration: Ox. ac.
Faintness: Dulc.
Fear of being alone: Ars.
—— —— —— touched: Iod.
—— —— death: *Acon. Ars.* Raph. Sec.
—— —— strangers: Bar. c. Caust.
Fitful mood: Nux mos.
Fretting: Psor.
Homesickness: Caps.
Hopelessness: *Psor.*
Hurry, does everything in a: Sul. ac.
——, feeling of : Lil. tig.
Hysterical mood: Asaf. Ign.
Imagination that another person is sick: *Petrol.*
—— —— body is broken into pieces: *Bapt.*
—— —— one is double: *Bapt.*
Imbecility, idiocy: Bar. c.
Impatience: Carbol. ac.
Impertinence: Graph.
Inability to perform tasks, feeling of: Lil. tig.
Indifference: China, Crotal. *Jatr.* Merc. v. *Phos. ac.* Picric ac. Rhod.
Intoxication: Gels.
Irritability, ill humor: Æscul. Æth. Alum. Amm. m. Ant. t. Ars. Asaf. Bell. Bol. *Bry.* Calc. c. Calc. ph. Canth. Carbo v. *Cham.* Cicuta, *Cina*, Colch. Colost. Dulc. Hep. Hydroph. *Iod*. Ipec. Kali bich. Kali c. Kreos. Lyc. Mur. ac. Natr. c. Natr. mur. Nitr. ac. Nuph. *Nux v.* Petrol. Phos. Plant. Psor.

Puls. Rheum, Staph. Sulph. *Sul ac.*
Large, things seem too: Hyos.
Laugh, tendency to: Nux mos.
Loquacity: Lach. Rhus, Stram.
Memory, loss of: Fluor. ac.
——, **weak:** Bar. c. Caust.
Moaning: Cham.
——, **continuously:** Carbol. ac.
Moroseness: Agar.
Obstinacy: *Calc. c.* Sil. Sulph.
Over-sensitiveness: *Coff.* Colch. *Nux v.* Phos. Samb. Staph.
Peevish, tearful: Ferr.
Petulance: Carbol. ac.
Repeats things said: Zinc.
Self-will: Agar.
Sentimental Mood: Ant. c.
Seriousness: Alum.
Sinking through the bed, sensation as if: Rhus.
—— **with bed, and everything in room, sensation as if:** Lach.
Slowness in learning to walk and talk: Agar.
Startled easily: Bell. *Bor.* Caust. Kali c.
Strikes and bites: *Stram.*
Stubbornness: Agar.
Stupidity: Bar. c.
Thought, vanishing of: Apis, Nitr. ac. Plant.
——, **wandering of:** Apis.
Time seems to pass slowly: Arg. n.
Whining restlessness: Cham.

Wilfulness: Calc. c.
Will power, lack of: Picric ac.

2. Head.

Bones, cranial, soft and thin: *Calc. ph.*
Fontanelles, open: Apis, **Calc. c. Calc. ph.** Ipec. *Merc. v.* Sep. **Sil. Sulph.**
——, anterior, large and sunken: *Apis.*
——, posterior, very large: *Calc. ph.*
——, sunken: *Apis*, Calc. c.
Hair, dry: Calc. c.
——, ——, rapidly falling off, with much dandruff: *Kali c.*
Headache: Æscul. *Aloe*, Ant. t. Asclep. Bol. *Calc. ph.* Cicuta, Cyclam. Hip. m. Iod. Iris v. Jabor. Kali nit. *Natr. mur.* Petrol. Picric ac. Plant. Podo. Rhus, Rum. Sabad. Tereb.
——, alternating with diarrhœa: Podo.
Head, automatic motion of: *Hell.* Zinc.
——, boring of, into pillow: *Apis, Bell. Bry.*
——, congestion to: Ferr. Graph.
—— drawn to one side: Stram.
——, dropping and raising of, spasmodic: Stram.
——, dulness of: Asar. E. Corn. c. Nitr. ac. *Nux v.*
—— hot: Apis, Arn. *Bell.* Bor. Bry. Hell. Kali brom.
——, ——, at occiput: Bell. *Zinc.*
——, ——, —— ——, forehead cool: *Zinc.*
——, ——, with cold hands and feet: **Bell.**

Head feels scattered about the bed: Bapt.

——, fore- cold, becomes warm if lightly covered: Sil.

——, ——, pain in: Apis, Arg. nit.

——, jerking backward and forward of: Sep.

——, —— —— of, violent: Cicuta.

——, large: *Calc. c. Calc. ph.* Merc. v. *Sil.*

——, pressure: Asar. E.

——, rheumatic pains in: Acon. Cham.

——, rolling of: *Bell.* Bry. *Hell.* Kali brom. *Podo.* Sil. Stram. *Zinc.*

——, —— ——, with moaning: Lyc.

——, sweat on: *Calc. c. Calc. ph.* Cham. *Sil.*

——, —— ——, when sleeping: **Calc. c.** *Calc. ph. Merc. v.* Podo. *Sil.*

——, —— ——, cold: Benz. ac.

——, —— ——, oily, offensive: *Merc. v.*

——, —— ——, sour-smelling: *Merc. v.* Sil.

——, —— —— forehead: Ant. t. Stann.

——, —— —— ——, cold: China, *Ipec.* **Verat.**

——, —— —— ——, ——, when sleeping: *Merc. v. Sil.*

——, —— —— ——, warm: Crot. tig.

——, tossing of hands to: Bry.

——, vise, feeling as though were in: Æth.

Vertigo: Acon. Agar. Alum. Arg. n. Camph. China, Cicuta, Crot. tig. Cyclam. Hip. m. Kali bich. Merc. v. Tabac. Tereb. Verat.

——, air, in open: Agar.

——, bed, when turning in: *Con.*

——, eating, after: Puls.

Vertigo, lying, when: *Con.*
——, **morning, in:** Agar.
——, **rising, when:** *Acon.*
——, **stooping, when:** Puls.
——, **sun, in bright:** Agar.
——, **vomiting, when:** Crot. tig.

3. Eyes and Ears.

Ears, ringing in: *China.*
Eyes, blue rings around: Ars. Bis. Calc. ph. Corn. c. Cupr. Cyclam. Ign. Ipec. Jatr. Lyc. Oleand. Phos. Rhus, Sec. Staph. Sulph.
——, **burning in:** Rhod.
——, **congested:** *Bell.* Kali brom.
——, **dim, dull:** Ant. t. Merc. v.
——, **distorted:** Bell.
——, **fixed:** Bry. *Camph.* Lyc. Zinc.
——, **half-open:** Bell. Hell. Podo. Sulph.
——, **itching voluptuous, of canthi and lids:** Gamb.
——, **motion of, convulsive:** Kali brom.
——, **moving in every direction without taking any notice:** Kali brom.
——, **pains in:** Apis.
——, **pupils contracted:** Cyclam. *Op. Verat.*
——, —— **dilated:** Arg. n. **Bell.** Calc. c. China, Cicuta, Cyclam. Hell. Hyos. Ipec. Kali brom. Laur. Picric ac.
——, **reddish tint:** Apis.
——, **rolled upward:** Apis, Cicuta, Hell.
——, **staring:** Bry. Cicuta, Hyos. Laur. Zinc.

Eyes, strabismus: *Alum*. Cina, Hell. Stram. Zinc.
——, **sunken:** *Camph*. Cupr. Iris v. Kali brom. Phos. Puls. Sec. Sep. Stann. Verat.
——, **swelling over:** *Kali c.*
——, **winking, absence of:** *Lyc.*
——, **yellow:** *Chel*. Con. Corn. c. *Dig*. Nux v.

4. Nose.

Nose, bleeding of, with pale face: Ipec.
——, **blueness around:** Kreos.
——, **boring in:** *Cina*, Zinc.
——, **paleness around:** *Cina*.
——, **picking of:** *Cina*.
——, **small scabs on septum of:** *Kali bich*.
Nostrils sore, cracked and crusty: *Ant. c.*

5. Face.

Cheeks red: Amm. m. Caps. Cham. Ferr.
——, **one hot, the other cold:** Kali c.
——, **one red, the other pale:** *Cham*.
Expression of anguish: Æth. *Canth*. Cupr.
—— —— **exhaustion:** Raph.
—— —— **pain:** Raph.
—— —— **terror and imbecility:** Acon.
——, **wretched:** Mez.
Face, acne, itching violently: Caust.
——, **altered:** Æth. Cupr.
——, **besotted look:** *Bapt*.
——, **bloated:** Bar c. Calc. c. China, Puls.

Face, bluish: Acon. *Camph.* **Cupr.** Dig. Kali brom. *Verat.*
——, brown: Arg. n.
——, changeable color: Phos.
——, cold: Ars. Bell. Calc. c. *Camph.* Cupr. Verat.
——, collapsed: Æth. *Camph.*
——, deathlike: Ars. *Canth.* Verat.
——, distorted: Ars. *Camph.* Cupr. Sec.
——, dull: Corn. c. Merc. v.
——, earthy: Ars. Bor. China, Lyc. Merc. v. Mez. Nux v. Op. Sil.
——, eruption on, red: Bor.
——, flushed: *Acon.* Æth. Amm. m. Bapt. Bar. c. *Bell.* Bol. Calc. c. Caps. Cicuta, Ferr. Hyos. Ign. Jabor. Lyc. Merc. v. Mur. ac. Nux v. Phos. Stann. Tereb. Zinc.
——, ——, dark red: *Bapt. Op.*
—— ——, when lying: *Acon.*
——, gray: Laur. Mez.
——, greasy-looking: *Natr. mur.*
——, greenish: Carbo v.
——, heat in: Corn. c. Op.
——, hippocratic: Acon. Hell.
——, livid: *Camph.* Laur.
——, pale: Ant. c. Ant. t. Apis, Arg. Arn. Ars. Bell. Bis. Bor. Calc. c. Calc. ph. *Camph. Canth. Carbo v.* China, Cicuta, Cina, Colch. Colost. Con. *Cupr.* Cyclam. Dig. Dulc. Ferr. Hell. Ign. Iod. *Ipec.* Jatr. Kali bich. Kali brom. Merc. v. Mez. Mur. ac. Natr. mur.

Nitr. ac. Nuph. Nux v. Oleand. Op. Phos.
Phos. ac. Plumb. Psor. Puls. Rheum, Rhus,
Sec. Sep. Sil. Stann. Staph. Stram. Sulph.

Face, pale around the nose and mouth: *Cina*.
— , — , when rising: *Acon*.
— , sallow: Arg. n. Calc. ph. Caust. Con. *Lept*.
Merc. v. Plumb. *Sep*. Sulph.
— , sickly: Phos. ac. Psor. Stann. Staph.
— , sunken: Ant. t. Apis, Arg. n. Arn. Calc.
c. Calc. ph. Corn. c. Ign. Laur. Mur. ac.
Oleand. Op. Rhus, Sec. Sep. Staph.
— , sweat on, cold: Ars. *Camph*. Sulph.
— , — — , cool: Rheum.
— , — — , when eating: Sul. ac.
— , swollen: Apis, Hell. Kali c. Op.
— , twitching of: Ipec.
— , yellowish: Ars. Corn. c. *Dig*. Iod. Kali
bich. Kali c. Laur. Merc. v. Nitr. ac. Nux
v. Sarsap. Sep.
— , yellow saddle aross nose: *Sep*.
— , waxy: Apis, Ars.
— , wrinkled: Arg. n. Calc. c. Psor. *Sarsap*.

Lips, black: Acon. Ars. Rhus, Verat.
— , blue: Ars. Carbo v. *Cupr*. Verat.
— , cold: Ars. Cupr. Verat.
— , cracked: Ars. Bry. Caps.
— , dark: Acon. Ars. Rhus.
— , dry: Acon. Arg. n. Ars. *Bry*. China, Crot.
tig. Rhus, Verat. *Zinc*.
— , pulling at: *Zinc*.
— , red: Aloe, *Sulph*.

Lips, swollen: Bry. Caps.
———, ———, upper: *Calc. c.* Natr. mur.
———, ulcers and blisters on: Nitr. ac.

6. MOUTH.

Aphthæ: Æth. Ars. Bapt. *Bor.* Calc. c. Canth. Caps. Corn. c. Dulc. Gamb. Hell. Hip. m. Iod. Kali brom. Magn. c. Merc. c. *Merc. v. Mur. ac.* Natr. mur. Nitr. ac. *Sarsap.* Sep. Staph. *Sulph. Sul. ac.*
Chewing motion: Bell. *Stram.*
Gums, bleeding: Arg. n. Bapt. Carbo v. Merc. v. Nux v. Phos. ac. Plant. Staph. Zinc.
———, sore: Arg. n. Bol. Gels.
———, spongy: Dulc. *Merc. v.* Natr. mur. Nitr. ac. *Staph.*
———, swollen: Calc. c. Cham. Gels. Kreos. *Merc. v.* Nux v. Phos. ac.
Gums, swollen, looking as if infiltrated with a dark watery fluid: *Kreos.*
Mouth, bleeding from: Bor. Hip. m.
———, burning from, to anus: Iris v.
———, ———, in: Asaf. Hip. m. *Iris v.* Jatr. Tarax.
———, coated white with clean, dark red, sensitive patches: *Tarax.*
———, corners of, sore, cracked and crusty: *Ant c.* Natr. mur.
———, distorted: Bell.
———, dry: Æscul. Asaf. Bell. Bry. Calc. c. Calc. ph. Canth. Cham. Cupr. Hip. m. Jatr. Kali

bich. Kali brom. Mur. ac. Natr. mur. Nux
mos. Op. Puls. Rum. Sec.

Mouth, frothy mucus in: Phos ac.

——, **hot:** *Bor.* Colch.

——, **open:** Bell.

——, **rawness from, to stomach:** *Tarax.*

——, —— **in:** *Tarax.*

——, **smarting in:** *Tarax.*

——, **sore:** Bapt. *Canth.* Dig.

——, **spits fluid out of, or squirts it across the bed:** Bapt.

——, **thrush in:** Kali brom.

——, **vesicles about:** *Natr. mur.*

——, **viscid mucus in:** *Natr. mur. Phos. ac.* *Puls.* Scill.

Palate wrinkled: Bor.

Saliva, bitter: Kali bich.

——, **bloody:** Ars.

——, **fetid:** *Dig.* Hip. m. Petrol.

——, **frothy:** Kali bich.

——, **increased:** Ant. c. Bell. Calc. c. *Carbo v.* China, *Colch. Dig.* Dulc. Grat. Hell. Hip. m. Hydroph. Iod. Ipec. Iris v. **Jabor.** Jatr. Kali bich. **Merc. v.** Mez. Nitr. ac. *Puls.* Rheum, Rhus, Sabad. *Sang.* Sulph. Sul. ac. Verat. Zinc.

——, **like cotton:** Nux mos. Puls.

——, **oily:** Cub.

——, **salt:** Kali bich.

——. **soap-like:** Dulc.

——, **sour:** Tarax.

Saliva, stringy, ropy: Cupr. *Kali bich.* Tarax.

———, **sweetish:** Cupr. *Dig.*

———, **tough:** Tarax.

———, **yellowish:** Hip. m.

Smell from the mouth, fetid: Iod. Kali nit. Lyc. *Merc. v.* Nux v. Petrol. Podo. Puls. Sep.

——— ——— ——— ———, **like onions:** Petrol.

——— ——— ——— ———, **putrid:** Lyc. Nitr. ac. Petrol. Rhus.

Taste, bitter: Acon. Aloe, Amm. m. *Arn.* Ars. Bol. *Bry.* Cham. Chel. China, Coloc. Corn. c. Cyclam. Elat. Gamb. Graph. Hep. Hip. m. Iris v. *Kali c.* Lyc. Magn. c. Merc. v. Natr. c. Natr. s. Nitr. ac. Nux v. Petrol. Phos. Picric ac. *Puls.* Raph. Sabad. Sil. Sulph. Verat.

———, ———, **of everything except water:** Acon.

———, ———, **of food:** Asar. E. *Bry.* China, Rhus, Scill.

———, **chalky:** Nux mos.

———, **flat:** Bol. Caps. Ign. Iris v. Nux mos.

———, **fresh, of food:** Coccul.

———, **greasy:** Asaf.

———, **long after, of food:** *Puls.* Zinc.

———, **lost:** Bol. Cupr. Cyclam. *Natr. mur.* Puls. Sabad.

———, **metallic:** Bol. Chel. Coccul. Hep. Merc. c. Merc. v. Sarsap.

———, **nauseous:** Crotal.

———, **putrid:** *Arn. Caps.* Graph. Iris v. Merc. v

MOUTH

Nux v. Plant. Puls. Rhus, Sep. Sulph. Verat.

Taste, rancid: Carbo v.
——, **salt**: Nux mos. Phos.
——, ——, **of food**: Sep. Sulph.
——, **slimy**: Arn. Cham. Zing.
——, **sour**: Arn. Calc. c. Caps. Cham. Chel. China, Coccul. Graph. Hep. Iod. Lyc. Nitr. ac. Nux v. Petrol. Phos. Sep. Sulph. Verat.
——, ——, **of food**: Calc. c. Caps. Lyc.
——, **straw-like, of food**: Stram. Sulph.
——, **sweet**: Cupr. Nuph. Phos. Sabad. Sulph.
——, ——, **of food**: Scill.
——, **watery**: Caps.

Teeth decay as soon as they appear: Kreos. *Staph.*
—— —— **at the roots, the crowns remaining sound**: Thuja.
—— **exhibit dark red spots or streaks as soon as they appear**: Kreos. *Staph.*
——, **grinding of**: Bell. *Cina*, Plant. Tabac.
——, **painful**: Arg. n.
——, **sensitive**: Arg. n. Bol. *Merc. v.*
——, **too long, feeling**: *Merc. v.*

Tongue bloody: Lach.
——, **burning of**: Coloc. Gamb.
——, **catching of, when protruding**: *Apis, Lach.*
——, **clean**: Dig. Hyos. *Ipec.* Phos. *Rhus,* Sarsap.
——, **coated**: Graph. Iod. Kali bich.

Tongue, coated black: Ars. Lach. Merc. v.
——, —— **brown:** Ars. Bry. Kali bich. Rhus. Sulph.
——, —— **stripes, in:** Bell.
——, —— **thick:** Kali bich. Nux v. Raph. Sec.
——, —— **white:** Agar. *Ant. c. Bis.* Bol. Bry. Cham. Chel. China, Coloc. Colost. Corn. c. Cyclam. Dig. Gels. Iris v. Kali nit. Kreos. Laur. Magn. c. Merc. v. Nux v. Oleand. Petrol. Phos. Plant. Podo. *Puls.* Raph. Rhus, Sang. Sarsap. Sec. Sep. Verat. Zinc.
——, —— —— **with clean red spots:** Hip. m. Tarax.
——, —— —— —— **red tip:** Cyclam.
——, —— —— —— —— —— **and borders:** Sul.
——, —— **yellow:** Bol. Bry. Cham. China, Coloc. Colost. Corn. c. Gels. Lept. Merc. v. Mez. Nux v. Podo. Rhus, Rum. Sec. Stann. Verat.
——, —— —— **thick fur:** Carbol. ac.
——, —— **yellowish-brown in the centre, with red, shining edges:** *Bapt.*
—— —— —— **white:** Gels.
——, —— —— **with white centre:** Sabad.
——, **cold:** Camph. *Carbo v.* Cupr. Sec. Verat.
——, **cracked:** Ars. *Kali bich.* Phos. Rhus, Sulph. Verat.
——, —— **at tip:** *Lach.*
——, **dry:** Aloe, Apis, Ars. Bapt. Bell. Bry. Calc. ph. Carbol. ac. Cham. Dulc. Hyos.

Iod. *Kali bich*. Laur. Mur. ac. Phos. Podo. *Rhus*, Sec. Sulph. Verat.

Tongue fissured: Raph.
—— heavy: Mur. ac.
—— livid: Sec.
—— mapped: Kali bich. *Natr. mur*. Tarax.
—— moist: Bell. Phos.
—— pale reddish-blue: Raph.
—— red: Aloe, Bell. Bry. Coloc. *Kali bich* Lach. Rhus, *Tereb*. Verat.
—— —— on tip and edges: Bell.
—— rough: *Rhus*.
—— scalded: Coloc.
—— shining: Apis, *Lach*. Tereb.
—— shriveled: *Mur. ac.*
—— smooth: *Kali bich*. Lach.
——, slimy: Chel. Petrol. Phos. ac.
——, sore: Canth. Dig. Merc. c. Sabad. Tereb.
——, streak, red, dry, down the middle: *Phos*.
—— swollen: Merc. v.
—— ——, taking impressions of teeth: Bol. Merc. v.
——, trembling of: Lach. Merc. v.
——, triangular red tip of: Rhus.
——, vesicles at tip: *Lach*.
——, —— on: Cyclam.
——, —— —— borders: *Apis*.

7. THROAT.

Throat and larynx feel as if closed: Tarax.

Throat, dry: Æscul. Cicuta, Cist. Nitr. ac.
——, dryness in, after diarrhœa: Ox. ac.
——, glassy looking: Cist.
——, pressure at pit of stomach, as of a foreign body: Caust.
——, spasms of, preventing speech: Cupr.
——, stripes of tough mucus on back of: Cist.
Goitre: Cist.

8. ŒSOPHAGUS.

Œsophagus, burning in: Camph. Sabad.
——, constriction of, when swallowing: Alum. Colch. Laur.
——, reversed peristalsis of: Asaf.
——, sensation of a ball rising in: *Asaf.* Ign.
——, soreness of: *Asaf.*

9. APPETITE.

Appetite, canine: *Bar. c. Calc. c. Calc. ph.* Coloc. Ferr. *Iod.* Lyc. *Merc. v.* Natr. mur. Oleand. Phos. ac. *Psor.* Sabad. Sarsap. Sil. Stann. Staph. Sulph. Verat.
——, ——, after vomiting: Oleand.
——, ——, 10 to 11 A. M.: Sulph.
——, ——, 11 or 12 A. M.: Zinc.
——, ——, with headache, if not gratified: Lyc.
——, ——, with weakness, if not gratified: *Phos.*
——, ——, worse at night: China.
——, capricious: *Cina.*

Appetite, diminished or lost: Amm. m. Ant. t. Apis, *Arn.* Ars. Asaf. Asar. E. Bell. Bol. Bor. Canth. Chel. China, Cicuta, Colch. Colost. Cop. Dig. Dulc. Ferr. Fluor. ac. Gamb. Iris v. Kali nit. Laur. Lil. tig. Lith. c. Magn. c. Nicc. Nux mos. Nux v. Oleand. Paul. Plant. Podo. Psor. Puls. Rhus, Sang. Sec. Sil. Stann. Stram. Sulph. Thromb. Verat. Zing.

——, **evening, prevents sleep:** Ign.

——, **good:** *Aloe, Calc. c.* Hep. Sarsap.

——, **hunger, without:** Nicc.

Aversion to acids: Bell. Coccul. Ferr. Sabad.

—— —— **ale or beer:** Bell. Ferr. Nux v.

—— —— **bread:** Cyclam. Hip. m. Lil. tig. Lyc. *Natr. mur.* Nitr. ac. Nux v. Puls.

—— —— ——, **brown:** Kali c.

—— —— **broth:** Arn.

—— —— **cheese:** *Chel.* Oleand.

—— —— **coffee:** Fluor. ac. Lil. tig. Lyc. Natr. mur. Nux v. Sabad.

—— —— ——, **smell of:** Sul. ac.

—— —— **drinks:** Canth. Coccul. Samb.

—— —— **eggs:** Ferr.

—— —— **fish:** Graph.

—— —— **food:** Arn. Bell. Canth. Cham. Coccul. *Colch.* Ipec. Op. Sabad. Sil.

—— —— ——, **fat:** Cyclam. Merc. v. Petrol. *Puls.*

—— —— ——, **warm, boiled:** Lyc.

—— —— ——, ——, **cooked:** Ign. Petrol. **Sil.**

Aversion to fruit: Bar. c.

— — meat: Aloe. Alum. Arn. Bell. Ferr. *Graph.* Hip. m. Ign. Lyc. Merc. v. Mur. ac. Nitr. ac. Petrol. Puls. Sabad. Sep. *Sulph.*

— — —, boiled: *Chel.* Nitr. ac.

— — milk: Magn. c. Natr. c. Puls. Sep. Tart. e.

— — mother's milk: *Sil.*

— — nursing: Ant c.

— — salt things: Graph.

— — smoking: Brom. Grat. Lyc.

— — solids: Ang.

— — sour things: See **Aversion to acids.**

— — spirits: Hip. m. Ign.

— — sweets: Bar. c Caust. Graph. Nitr. ac.

— — tobacco: Canth. Coccul. Ign. Nux v.

— — water: Hydroph.

— — wine: Hip. m. Sabad.

Desire for acids: Alum. Ant. c. Ant. t. Arn. Ars. Bor. Brom. Bry. China, Cina, Cist. Cub. Dig. Hep. Kali bich. Kali c. Magn. c. Podo. Psor. *Verat.*

— — acid food: Cist.

— — almonds: Cub.

— — apples: Aloe.

— — bacon: *Calc. ph.*

— — beer or ale: Aloe, Kali bich. Merc. v. Puls. Sulph.

— — bitter things: Dig. *Natr. mur.*

— — brandy: Cub. Nux v. Sulph.

— — bread: Cub. Grat.

APPETITE.

Desire for butter: *Merc. v.*
— — chalk: Nitr. ac. Nux v.
— — charcoal: *Alum*. Cicuta.
— — cheese: Cist.
— — cherries: China.
— — chocolate: Hydroph.
— — cloves: Alum.
— — coffee: Bry. Caps. Carbo v. Con. Mez
— — —, ground, burned: Alum.
— — cold food or drink: Ant. t. Ars. Bell. Bry. **Phos** Rhus, Sil. *Verat.*
— — condiments: *Hep.*
— — dainties: Ipec.
— — delicacies: Cub.
— — earth: *Alum*. Nitr. ac.
— — eggs: *Calc. c.*
— — farinaceous food: Sabad.
— — fat food, *Calc. ph*. Merc. Nitr. ac. Nux v.
— — fluids only: Acet. ac.
— — fruit: Ant. t. China, Cist. Cub. Magn. c. *Verat.*
— — ham fat: Mez.
— — herring: Nitr. ac.
— — hot drinks: *Chel.* Cupr.
— — indigestible substances: Alum.
— — juicy things: Aloe, *Phos. ac.*
— — lemonade: Cyclam. Puls. *Sec.*
— — lime: Nitr. ac.
— — milk: Apis, Chel. Merc. v.
— — —, cold: *Rhus.*

Desire for nuts: Cub.
—— —— onions: Cub.
—— —— oranges: Cub.
—— —— oysters: Lach. *Natr. mur*. Rhus.
—— —— piquant things: Fluor. ac. Sang.
—— —— rags, clean: *Alum*.
—— —— refreshing, something: *Phos. ac.*
—— —— rice, dry: Alum.
—— —— salt: *Natr. mur*.
—— —— —— food: Calc. c. Calc. ph. Con. *Natr. mur*.
—— —— seasoned, highly, things: Fluor. ac. Hep.
—— —— smoked meats: **Calc. ph.** *Kreos*.
—— —— sour things: See **Desire for acids.**
—— —— spirits: Arn. Ars. Cupr. Puls.
—— —— starch: Alum. Nitr. ac.
—— —— sugar: **Arg. n.** Kali c.
—— —— sweet things: Calc. c. Ipec. Lyc. Sabad.
—— —— tea: Hep.
—— —— —— grounds: Alum.
—— —— various things, becoming repugnant when little is eaten: *Rheum*.
—— —— warm drinks only: Ang.
—— —— —— food: Cupr.
—— —— wine: Ars. Bry. Calc. c. Chel. China, Cub. Hep. Lach. Mez. Sulph.

Thirst: Aloe, Ant. c. Ant. t. Arn. Bapt. Calc. c. Calc. ph. Carbol. ac. Caust. Cham. China, Cicuta, Coccul. *Colch*. Coloch. Corn. c. Cy-

clam. Dig. Dulc. Hell. Hep. Hip. m. Hyos.
Iod. Kali bich. Kali nit. Lach. Laur. Magn.
c. Merc. v. Mez. Natr. c. Natr. mur. Nicc.
Nitr. ac. *Nux v.* Oleand. *Phos.* Phos. ac.
Picric ac. Plant. Podo. *Rhus*, Samb. Scill.
Sil. Stram. Sulph. Thuja, *Verat.* Zing.

Thirst, burning: *Ars.* Canth. Colch. Jabor.

——, **constant:** Æth. *Ars.* Bel. Calc. c. Cham. Sulph. Tabac.

——, **drink descending with gurgling:** Cupr. *Laur.* Thuja.

——, **drinking large quantities:** *Bis.* Stram. *Verat.*

——, —— —— —— **at long intervals:** Bry.

——, —— **small quantities often:** Ant. t. Apis, **Ars.** Bell. China.

——, **evening, in the:** *Natr. mur. Natr. s.*

——, **intense:** Acet. ac.

——, **morning, in the:** Nitr. ac. Sep.

——, **night, at:** Ant. c. Calc. c. Phos. Rhus.

—— **unquenchable:** **Acon.** *Ars.* Camph. Canth. Colch. Cub. Cupr. Ferr. Grat. *Jatr. Verat.*

——, **vomiting after:** Oleand.

——, **with nausea:** Bapt.

——, **without desire for drink:** Ang. Graph.

Thirstlessness: Ant. c. Ant. t. **Apis,** Arg. n. Bapt. Camph. Canth. Caps. *Cyclam.* Ferr. *Gels.* Ipec. Lyc. Nux mos. Podo. **Puls.** Sarsap. Staph.

—— **in croup:** Acet. ac.

10. Eructations.

Eructations: Ant. c. Bell. *Carbo v.* China, Cyclam. Diosc. Dulc. Ipec. Iris v. Lach. Lyc. Plant. Rum. Zing.
—, **bitter:** Amm. m. Cham. Ign.
—, **carried, when:** Kreos.
—, **difficult, causing strangulation:** *Arg. n.*
—, **enormous:** Iris v.
—, **fetid:** Ant. t. Arn. Asaf. Carbo v. Graph. Psor. Sep.
—, **forcible:** Iris v.
—, **loud:** *Arg. n. Carbo v.*
—, **rancid:** Asaf. *Carbo v. Graph.* Sabad.
—, **smelling like rotten eggs:** *Ant. t. Psor.*
—, **sour:** Arn. Hep. Kali c. Natr. c. Natr. s. Picric ac. Podo. Sabad. Sil. Sulph. Zing.
—, —— **water:** *Nicc.*
—, **tasting of food:** Ant. c.
Hiccough: Æth. Carbo v. Cicuta, *Hyos. Ign.* Jabor. Nux v. Tabac.
—, **carried when:** *Kreos.*

11. Nausea and Vomiting.

Nausea: Ant. t. Apis, *Arg. n.* Arn. Ars. Bapt. Bell. Bis. Bol. Bov. Brom. Camph. Cicuta, Cist. Coccul. *Colch. Coloc.* Con. Cop. Corn. c. *Crot. tig.* Cub. Cyclam. Dig. Diosc. Dulc. Gamb. Grat. Hep. Ign. *Ipec.* Iris v. Jabor. Jalap. Lept. Lyc. Merc. v. Mur. ac. Natr. mur. Nicc. Nitr. ac. Nux v. Oleand. Op.

Petrol. Plant. Plumb. Podo. Raph. Rheum,
Rhus, Rum. Sabad. Sang. Sarsap. Scill. Sec.
Sep. Sil. Stann. *Sulph*. *Tabac*. *Verat*. Zinc.
Zing.

Nausea, with gagging (retching): *Ant. t.* Arn.
Asar. E. *Bell*. **Bis**. Bry. China, Coloc. Crot.
t. Hell. Ign. *Ipec*. Jabor. *Kreos*. Nux v. *Podo*.
Puls. *Sec*. Verat.

——, after fresh meat: *Caust.*

——, mornings: Ang.

——, on rising: **Bry**. Picric ac.

——, on seeing food: Ars. *Colch.*

——, on smelling food: Colch. *Stann.*

——, —— —— broth: Colch.

——, —— —— eggs: Colch.

——, —— —— fat meat: Colch.

——, —— —— fish: Colch.

——, relieved by a soft stool: Tereb.

——, with hunger: Ign.

——, —— pale face and suppressed breathing: Ipec.

——, —— thirst: Bapt.

Vomiting: Acon. Æth. *Ant. c.* Ant. t. Arn. *Ars*.
Bapt. Bell. Bry. Camph. Carbo v. Carbol. ac.
Cicuta, *Coccul*. Coloc. Cop. Crotal. Diosc.
Elat Ferr. Gamb. Hip. m. Iod. *Ipec. Iris v.*
Jabor. Jalap. Kali bich. Kreos. Lept. Merc.
v. Mur. ac. Natr. mur. Petrol. Plumb.
Sabad. Sarsap. Scill. *Sec.* Sep. *Sulph. Verat.*

——, acrid: Ferr. Hep. *Iris v.*

——, albuminous substance: Merc. c.

Vomiting, as soon as stomach is full: *Bis.*
——, bilious: Acon. *Ant. c.* Apis, Ars. China, Coloc. Cupr. Dig. Elat. Fluor. ac. Ipec. Iris v. Jatr. Kali bich. Podo. Puls. Raph. Sec. Stram. Verat.
——, bitter: Ant. c. Apis. Bol. Bry. Colch. Colost. Grat. Hip. m. Kali bich. Puls. Sang.
——, black substances: Ars. Hell.
——, bloody: Acon. Ars. Kali bich.
——, brown substances: Ars.
——, cold, when becoming: Coccul.
——, ——, food or drink, better after: **Phos.**
——, constant, with painless diarrhœa: Bor.
——, difficult: Ant. t.
——, drunk, of what has been: Acon. Ant. c. Arn. Ars. Bis. Sil. Verat.
——, ——, —— —— ——, as soon as it becomes warm: **Phos.**
——, ——, —— —— —— ——, immediately: Ars. Bis. Crot. tig. Ipec. *Zinc.*
——, easy: *Colch.* Sec.
——, eaten, of what has been: *Ant. c.* Ant. t. Ars. Cham. China, Coloc. Crot. tig. Dig. Ferr. Hep. Hip. m. *Ipec.* Iris v. Kali bich. Puls. Raph. Verat.
——, ——, —— —— —— ——, immediately: **Ars.** Ipec. *Sec.*
——, ——, —— —— —— ——, sour: *Calc. c. Hep.* Kali bich. Oleand. Podo. *Puls.* Sulph.
——, fluid, dark olive-green or black: Carbol. ac.

NAUSEA AND VOMITING.

Vomiting, ——, glairy: Kali bich.
——, ——, pinkish: Kali bich.
——, efforts to, violent, resulting in enormous forcible eructations: Iris v.
——, food, eaten hours before: *Kreos.*
——, frothy: Æth. Ant. t. Crot. tig. *Verat.*
——, ——, milky-white: Æth.
——, green, bitter substance: Merc. c.
——, greenish: Æth. Ant. c. Ant. t. Arg. n. Asar. E. Coloc. Dig. Hell. Hep. Hip. m. Jatr. Oleand. *Sec.* Stram.
——, —— watery, later colorless: Grat.
——, hot: Podo.
——, lying on left side, worse: Ant. t.
——, lying on right side, better: Ant. t.
—— milk: Æth. Arg. n. Calc. ph.
——, ——, of curdled: Æth. Ant. c. Calc. c.
——, ——, —— ——, in large lumps: Æth.
——, ——, mother's: *Sil.*
——, —— ——, if mother has been angry: Valer.
——, ——, soured: *Calc. c.*
——, mucus, of: Acon. Ant. c. Cyclam. Dig. Dulc. *Ipec.* Kali bich. Oleand. Puls. Sec.
——, ——, albuminous: *Jatr.*
——, ——, fetid: Ipec. *Sec.*
——, ——, frothy: Ant. t. Podo.
——, ——, glassy: Arg. n. Ars.
——, ——, green: Æth. Ars. Bry. *Ipec.* Podo. Verat.
——, ——, **jelly-like**: *Ipec.*

Vomiting, mucus, slimy: Bor. Cham.
——, ——, **stringy, tough:** Merc. c.
——, ——, **tenacious:** Arg. n. Dulc. Kali bich.
——, ——, **white:** Raph.
——, ——, **yellowish:** Ars. Bry. Colch. Ipec. Verat.
——, **oily:** Æth.
——, **persistent, after nausea ceases:** *Ant. c.*
——, **riding, when:** Coccul. Petrol.
——, **scanty:** Asar. E.
——, **sleep, after:** Æth. Cupr.
——, ——, **and exhaustion, after:** *Æth.*
——, **solids only, liquids retained:** *Bapt.*
——, **sour:** Ant. c. Apis, Asar. E. Bol. Bor. *Calc. c.* Cham. China, Colost. Ferr. Hep. *Iris v.* Kali c. Magn. c. Podo. *Puls.*
——, **violent, with pains in head:** Grat.
——, **water only, food is retained:** *Bis.*
——, **watery:** Ant. t. Bis. China, Crot. tig. Cupr. Grat. Hep. Hip. m. Oleand. Raph. Sang. Sec. Sulph. Tabac.
——, ——, **fat lumps, with:** *Hip. m.*
——, ——, **flakes, with:** Cupr.
——, ——, **greasy:** Hip. m.
——, ——, **greenish bilious matter, with great weakness:** Elat.
——, **with trembling of hands and fainting:** Ant. t.
——, **yellowish:** Grat.

12. STOMACH.

Stomach, acrid feeling in: Hep.

STOMACH.

Stomach, burning in: *Ars.* Bis. Camph. Cham. Cicuta, *Colch.* Crot. tig. Jatr. Sabad. *Sec.* Tabac.

———, ——— ———, **great:** Iris v.

———, **chilled easily by cold water:** Sul. ac.

———, **coldness in:** Caps. *Colch.* Grat.

———, **cold stone, feeling of, in:** Acon.

———, **contractions in, painful:** Æth.

———, **desire to loosen clothing about:** *Hep. Lach. Lyc.* Merc. c. *Nux v.*

———, ——— ——— **tighten clothing about:** Fluor. ac. *Natr. mur.*

———, **distension of:** *Lyc.* Merc. c. Natr. c.

———, **distress in:** Fluor. ac. Jabor. Natr. mur.

———, **empty feeling at:** Petrol. Phos. *Sep.* Stann. *Sulph.*

———, **faintness at:** Alum. Asaf. Bol. Brom. Hep. Sang.

———, ——— ——— **about 10 or 11 A. M.:** Lach. Mur. ac. Natr. c. **Sulph.**

———, **fulness of:** Arn. Bar. c. Cyclam. *Lyc.* Nux mos.

———, **gnawing at:** *Lith. c.* Natr. c. Sil.

———, **pains in:** Ars. Brom. Cist. Coccul. Coloc. Corn. c. Cupr. Elat. Iod. Jatr. *Lyc.* Staph. Zing.

———, **pressure at:** Bis. Camph. Caust. Crot. tig. Elat. Hep. Natr. c. Petrol. Picric ac. Scill. Verat.

———, **pulsations in:** Asaf.

———, **rawness from, to mouth:** *Tarax.*

Stomach, relaxed sensation in: *Staph.*
——, **sick feeling at**: Ipec.
——, **sinking at**: Bapt. *Dig. Hep. Ign.* Lyc. Nux v. Plant. *Sep. Sulph.*
——, **softening of**: Calc. c. Kreos.
——, **soreness in**: Merc. c. Nux mos.
——, **spasm of**: Brom. *Coccul. Cupr.* Jatr.
——, **tenderness**: Camph. Elat. *Lyc.* Ox. ac.

13. ABDOMEN.

Abdomen, burning in: Apis, Arg. n. *Ars.* Canth. Carbo v. Colch. Sarsap. Sec.
——, **cold**: Arn. Merc. v.
——, **coldness in**: Colch. *Grat.* Kali brom. Petrol. Sarsap. Sec. Tabac.
——, **colic**: Æscul. Aloe, Alum. Arg. n. Asaf. Bov. Bry. Calc. ph. Camph. Cantn. *China,* Cicuta, Coccul. Coff. Colch. *Coloc.* Crot. tig. Cub. *Cupr. Diosc.* Gamb. *Ipec.* Iris v. Kali bich. Kali brom. Kali nit. Lach. Laur. Merc. v. Natr. c. Natr. s. Nux v. Ox. ac. Petrol. Podo. Puls. Rhus, Sec. Stann. Tereb. *Thromb.* Verat.
——, —— **and backache at same time**: *Sarsap.*
——, ——, **cutting**: Acon. Ant. c. Arn. Bell. Cham. *China,* Cina, *Coloc.* Con. Cub. Dulc. Elat. Iod. *Jalap.* Lept. Magn. c. Mez. Nitr. ac. Nux v. Plumb. Rheum, Rhus, Sabad. Scill. Sulph.
——, ——, **griping**: Aloe, Coloc. Con. Corn. c.

ABDOMEN. 285

Ipec. Jalap. Kreos. Nux v. Plant. Samb. Thromb.

Abdomen, colic, pinching: Amm. m. Bor. China, Cina, Dulc. Ipec. Magn. c. Mez. Nux v. Petrol. Rhus, Sulph.

——, ——, **tearing:** Bell. Cham. Cicuta, Rhus.

——, ——, **twisting:** Diosc.

——, ——, **violent, flatulent, following an obstinate diarrhœa:** Elat.

——, **constriction of:** Arg. n. Bell. *Plumb.* Sabad.

——, **cramps in:** *Cupr.* Grat.

——, **cramp-like pains in:** Lach.

——, **distended (tympanitic):** Acon. Aloe, Apis, Arn. *Ars.* Asaf. Bar. c. Bell. Bis. Bor. Bov. *Calc. c.* Caps. *Carbo v.* Cham. Caust. *China,* Cicuta, Coff. Colch. Coloc. Con. Corn. c. Crot. tig. Cub. Cupr. *Graph.* Hip. m. Iris v. Jatr. Kali bich. Kali c. Kreos. Lach. Lil. tig. *Lyc.* Magn. c. Merc. c. Natr. mur. Nicc. *Nux mos.* Petrol. Phos. Phos. ac. Plant. Samb. *Sil.* Stram. **Tereb.**

——, **distress in:** Bol. *Lept.*

——, **empty or sick feeling:** Ferr. Jabor. *Petrol.* Phos. Plant. Podo. Sarsap.

——, **feeling as if bowels were falling out:** Kali brom.

——, **fermentation in:** *Arn.* China, *Lyc.* Phos. ac. Rhus, Sarsap.

——, **fulness in:** Acon. Aloe, Bell. Cyclam. Graph. *Lyc.* Natr. s. Sec.

Abdomen, gurgling in: *Aloe*, Asar. E. Gamb. *Jatr*. Zinc.

——, **hardness of:** Graph. *Sil*. Stram.

——, **heat in:** Aloe, Lach. Podo. *Sil*.

——, **hot, body cold:** Tabac.

——, **pains in:** Bapt.

——, ——, **aggravated from warm milk:** Ang.

——, —— **suddenly shift and appear in distant parts:** *Diosc*.

——, **pressure in:** Aloe, Cupr. Samb. Zinc.

——, **protrusion of intestines like pads, here and there:** Raph.

——, **retracted:** *Plumb*. Podo. Verat.

——, **retraction, feeling of, in:** Zinc.

——, **rumbling:** Æscul. Aloe, Ang. Arn. Asar. E. Bov. Calc. ph. Coccul. Coloc. Corn. c. Cyclam. Gamb. Iris v. Jatr. *Lyc*. Magn. c. Nitr. ac. Oleand. Phos. ac. Picric ac. Plant. Puls. Rhod. Sabad. Sarsap. Sec. Sil. Zinc. Zing.

——, —— **during and after drinking:** Phos.

——, **sensation of a ball moving and turning in:** Sabad.

——, —— —— **sharp stones rubbing together in:** Coccul.

——, **sensitive:** Acon. Aloe, **Apis**, Arg. n. Bell. Canth. Coff. *Coloc*. Crot. tig. Cub. Cupr. Cyclam. Ferr. Gamb. Kali c. Kreos. *Lach*. Lil. tig. Lyc. Merc. c. Natr. s. Nux v. Ox. ac. Phos. Tereb. Thromb. Verat

——, —— **over transverse colon:** Carbol. ac.

Abdomen, soreness in: Bapt.

———, **spasms of, with hardening of abdomen:** Kali brom.

———, **stitches in:** Arg. n. Kali c.

———, **sunken:** Bor. *Calc. ph.* Natr. mur.

———, **sunken, sensation as if:** Sabad.

———, **swollen:** Acet. ac.

———, **trembling sensation in:** Lil. tig.

———, **weight in:** Ferr.

Flatus: Amm. m. Bov. *Carbo v. China,* Cub. Grat. Kali c. Lach. *Natr. s. Nicc.* Nitr. ac. Nux v. Oleand. Phos. ac Sabad. Sep. Sil. Zing.

———, **cold:** Con.

——— **emission, of no:** Raph.

———, **fetid:** Arn. China, Coccul. Con. Natr. c. *Natr. s. Nicc.* Oleand. Petrol. Plant. Psor. Rhod. Sarsap. Scill. Staph. Sulph.

———, **garlic, smelling like:** *Agar.*

———, **hot:** Coccul. Staph.

———, **incarcerated:** *Lyc. Natr. s.* Sil.

———, ——— **at night in right abdomen:** Natr. s.

———, **in left abdomen:** Iod.

———, **offensive:** Aloe, Ang. Lith. c. Phos. Sang. Sep. Sil.

———, **putrid:** Carbo v. Oleand.

———, **sour:** Natr. c.

Hypochondria sensitive to pressure: Arg. n. Caust. Tabac.

Hypochondrium, pain in right: Bapt. Bol Merc. v. Natr. s.

Hypochondrium, pain in right, coughing, when: Psor.

——, —— —— ——, drinking cold water, when: Lept.

——, —— —— ——, laughing, when: Psor.

——, —— —— ——, lying on it, when: Psor.

——, —— —— ——, pressure by: Fluoric ac. Merc. v. Psor.

——, —— —— ——, stitching: *Kali c.* Sabad.

——, —— —— ——, walking, when: Natr. s. Psor.

——, —— ——, left, when drinking cold water: Natr. c.

Liver, indurated: Laur.

——, swollen: *China*, Laur. Nux mos.

——, tender: Dig. *Natr. s.*

Sides, Stitches in the: Merc. c.

Spleen, swollen: *China*, Iod.

Urging to stool unsuccessful: Corn. c. Natr. s.

14. ANUS.

Anus, biting at: Dulc.

——, burning from, to mouth: Iris v.

——, ——, soreness and fulness of: Æscul.

——, burning, redness and itching in and around: Zing.

——, constantly open: Phos.

——, itching of: Æscul.

——, oozing from: *Apis*, Ox. ac. **Phos.** *Sep. Thromb.*

——, —— of fluid smelling like herring brine: *Calc. c.*

Anus, prolapsus of, during urination: Mur. ac.
—, rawness, smarting, soreness of: Apis.
—, secretion of yellowish-white mucus at: Ant. c.
—, spasmodic pains in: Ferr.
—, sphincter, sensation of weakness in: Alum.

Hæmorrhoids: *Æscul. Aloe, Brom.* Calc. ph. Diosc. Fluor. ac. Graph. Lach. *Mur. ac.* Phos. Zing.

Rectum, crawling in: Calc. c.
—, croup of: Brom.
—, cutting and pinching pain in: Aloe.
—, dryness of, excessive: *Æscul.*
—, fulness in, feeling of: *Æscul.*
—, heat and itching in: *Æscul.*
—, pressing, contracting, tickling in: Ang.
— pricking pains in: Nuph.
—, protrusion of: Crot. tig. Podo.
—, pustules at side of: Amm. m.
—, soreness, itching of: Amm. m.
—, swollen feeling of mucous membrane of: *Æscul.*
—, urging in, with crawling over the face: Ang.

15. URINE.

Dysuria: Rheum.
Strangury: Ant. t. *Apis*, **Canth.** *Caps.* Coloc. Lil. tig. **Merc. c.** Merc. v. Nux v. Sulph. *Tereb.*

GENERAL ACCOMPANIMENTS.

Tenesmus of bladder: Arn. **Merc.** c. Merc. v.
Ureters, pain extending down: *Tereb.*
Urination, burning after: **Canth.** Iris v.
——, —— during: Tereb.
——, difficult: *Calc. c.* Caps. Nux v. Zinc.
——, flow interrupted: *Con.*
——, frequent: Acon. Ant. c. Apis, Bell. Bor. Canth. Coloc. *Con.* Dig. Lil. tig. Merc. v. Nux v. Phos. ac. Plant.
——, involuntary: Aloe, Bell. Caust. Cham. Hyos. Kreos. Merc. v. Natr. mur. Plant. Sep. Sil.
——, involuntary, at night, from laxity of sphincter vesicæ: *Plant.*
——, pain in bladder, after: *Lith. c.*
——, —— —— ——, before: *Lith. c.*
——, possible only with stool: **Alum.**
——, screaming before: *Bor. Lyc.*
——, —— during: Sarsap.
——, seldom: Cupr.
——, smarting during: *Lil. tig.*
——, urging, strong: Lith. c.
Urine, acrid: Bor. Merc. c. Merc. v.
——, albuminous: Tereb.
——, ammoniacal: Iod.
——, black: Carbol. ac.
——, blackish olive green: Carbol. ac.
——, bloody: Ant. t. *Merc. c. Tereb.* Zinc.
——, brown: Arn. Lept.
——, clear: *Acon. Bry.*
——, cloudy: Phos. ac. Tereb.

URINE. 291

Urine, dark: *Benz. ac.* Bol. Bry. Carbol. ac. China, Colch. Jabor. Nitr. ac. Rheum, Tereb.
———, ———, with floating black specks: Hell.
———, dribbling at beginning of stool: Kali brom.
———, excoriating: Sulph.
———, fetid: *Bapt.* Bor. *Calc. c.* Carbo v. Coloc. Graph. *Sep.* Tereb.
———, forming a white cloud on standing: Cina, *Phos. ac.*
———, frothy: *Lach.*
———, greenish: Ars. Chel.
———, hot: *Cham.* Merc. v.
———, jelly-like: *Cina,* Coloc.
———, liver-colored: Rheum.
———, muddy: Sabad.
———, onions, smelling like: Gamb.
———, pale: Chel. Phos. *Phos. ac.* Plant. Stann.
———, profuse: Aloe, Ant. c. Apis, Arg. n. Bell. Chel. Jabor. Merc. v. Ox. ac. Phos. Phos. ac Plant. Scill. Stann.
———, retained: *Ars.* Canth. Coloc. *Hyos.* Laur. Merc. c. Sulph. Verat.
———, scanty: Acon. Ant. t. *Arg. n.* Arn. Ars. Benz. ac. Bol. Colch. Cupr. Dig. Hell. Hyos. Jabor. Kali brom. Lil. tig. *Merc. c.* Merc. v. Nux mos. Op. Tereb.
———, smarting: Rheum.
———, sediment, coffee-grounds, like: *Hell.*
———, sediment, red: Ant. c. Graph. *Lyc.*

Natr. mur. *Sep.*

Urine, sediment red sand in streaks: Hyos.

——, ——, thick: *Bol.* Graph. Sep. Zinc.

——, ——, white sand: *Sarsap.*

——, ——, yeast-like: Raph.

——, ——, yellow: Zinc.

——, smoky: *Hell.* Tereb.

——, sour-smelling: Graph. Nitr. ac.

——, strong-smelling: *Benz. ac. Calc. c.* Nitr. ac.

——, suppressed: *Arg. n.* Ars. Bell. Canth. Carbo v. Crotal. Cupr. Laur. Lyc. *Merc. c.* Op. Podo. *Sec.* Sil. *Stram.* Sulph. Verat.

——, watery: Arg. n. Coccul. Ign. Phos. Phos. ac.

——, ——, inodorous with fetid stool of white mucus: Dulc.

——, white: *Cina,* Phos. ac. Stann.

——, yellow: Chel. Raph.

16. Sexual Organs.

Erections, priapismic: Picric ac.

Genitals, moist excoriation about: *Sulph.*

——, pulling at, constant: *Stram.*

Ovarian irritation: *Lil. tig.*

Prolapsus uteri: *Lil. tig.*

Sexual excitement: *Lil. tig.* Picric ac.

——, weakness: *Nuph.*

17. Chest.

Breath acrid-smelling (like horse radish): Agar.

CHEST.

Areath, cold: *Carbo v.*
——, **fetid:** *Arn.* Bapt. Caps. Gels. Mur. ac. Stann.
——, **offensive:** Nux mos.
Chest, burning in: Kali brom.
——, **constriction of:** Verat.
——, —— ——, **spasmodic:** Arg. n. Asaf. Cupr. Sec. Verat.
——, **oppression of:** Verat.
——, **stitches in:** *Bry. Kali c.*
——, **tonic spasms of:** Cicuta.
Cough, dry: Rum.
——, **followed by belching:** Sul. ac.
——, **loose, rattling, during dentition:** *Calc. c.*
Heart, beating of, not rapid, but too violent: Dig.
——, **irregular action of:** Laur.
——, —— —— ——, **with great cardiac anguish:** Laur.
——, —— —— ——, —— **suffocative attacks:** Laur.
——, **oppression of:** *Tabac.*
——, **palpitation of:** Ant. t. Cact. Cyclam.
——, —— ——, **with large and small beats intermingled:** Alum.
——, ——, **worse from least exertion:** Iod.
Respiration, difficult: Arg. n. Asaf. Elat. Puls.
——, ——, **when lifted from the cradle:** Calc. ph.
——, **feeble:** China, Laur.
——, **labored:** Apis, Arg. n. Carbo v. Cicuta,

Cupr.

Respiration, moaning: Laur.

———, oppressed: Crotal. Cupr. Ipec. Sulph. Tabac. Thuja, Verat.

———, rattling: *Op*

———, short: Thuja.

———, sighing: Arg. n. *Ign.*

———, slow: Laur.

———, snoring: *Op.*

Voice, choleraic: Ferr.

———, feeble: *Camph. Sec. Verat.*

———, hoarse: Camph. Carbo v. Sec. Verat.

———, hollow: Sec.

———, inaudible: Sec.

———, lost: *Carbo v.*

———, weak: Hell.

Yawning: Ant. t. Elat. Plant. Podo.

18. BACK AND NECK.

Back, aching of, relieved by pressure: *Natr. mur.*

———, ——— and colic at same time: *Sarsap.*

———, burning in: *Picric ac. Tereb.*

———, chills in: *Gels.*

———, coldness in: Sec.

———, dull, heavy pains in: Bol.

———, formication in: *Sec.*

———, lumbar region, painful soreness in: Bar. c.

———, renal region, dull pain and burning in: *Tereb.*

EXTREMITIES.

Back, renal region, sensitive to pressure: Tabac.
——, sacro-iliac symphysis, pains as if broken, in: Æscul.
——, sacro-lumbar region, aching in: Æscul.
——, sacrum, drawing, twisting pains in: Diosc.
——, scapula, pain under right: Chel.
——, scapulæ, burning between: Phos.
——, ——, heat between: Lyc.
——, small of, pain in: Bar. c.
——, spasmodic pains in: Ferr.
——, stitching pains in, extending into gluteal muscles: Kali c.
——, weakness and soreness of: Picric ac.
——, weight in, when standing: Arg. n.
Neck emaciation of: Natr. mur. Sarsap.
——, glands of, swollen: Iod.
——, rheumatic pains in: Acon.
——, slender: Calc. c. Calc. ph. Natr. mur.
Shoulders, rheumatic pains in: Acon.

19. EXTREMITIES.

Ankles weak: Calc. c. Calc. ph. Caust. Natr. c. Natr. mur. Sulph.
Arms and fingers, involuntary jerking of: Cicuta.
——, bruised feeling of: Cicuta.
——, cramps of: Cupr. Phos. ac. Verat.
——, fore-, icy coldness of: Apis, Brom. Colch.
Calves, cramps in: Merc. c.
Extremities and body, cold: Iris v.

Extremities, convulsive twitchings of: Kali brom. Stram.

——, cramps in: Hell.

——, icy coldness of: Sec.

Feet, blue: Kali brom.

——, cold: Bell. Carbo v. Kali brom. Kreos. *Lyc.* Nitr. ac. *Picric ac.* Puls. Sabad. Sec. Sil. Sulph.

——, constant motion of: Zinc.

——, drawing up the: Æth.

——, one hot, the other cold: Lyc.

——, soles of, hot: Sep. Sulph.

——, sweat of, offensive: Sil.

Fingers spread apart or bent backward: *Sec.*

Hands, blue: Apis, Kali brom.

——, cold: Apis, Kali brom. Kreos. Sulph.

——, cold, before vomiting: Verat.

——, ——, with warmth of body: Tabac.

——, ——, —— —— —— head: *Bell.*

——, cramps of: *Cupr.* Phos. ac. *Sec.* Verat.

——, hot, after vomiting: Verat.

——, ——, palms of: Bol. Bov. Phos. Sep. *Sulph.*

——, panaritium: Natr. s.

——, paronychia: Diosc.

——, sweat on, cold: Brom. Kali bich. Lil. tig.

——, warts on: Sarsap.

Legs, cold: Acon. Arn. *Calc. c.* Carbo. v. Cicuta, Colch. Merc. v. Sec. Sil. Tabac.

——, **cramps of:** Camph. Colch. *Cupr. Jatr. Podo. Sec.* Sulph. Tabac. Verat.

Legs, curvature of: Calc. c. *Calc. ph.*
——, debility felt mostly in. Arg. n.
——, formication in: *Sec.*
——, pains in: Bol. Diosc. *Rhus.*
——, paralytic feeling of: *Cocul.*
——, rheumatic pains in: Asclep. Merc. v.
——, swelling of: Acet. ac.
——, weakness of: Aloe, Arg. n. *Cocul.* Picric ac.

Nails, blue: Acon.

Shoulder, painful cutting jerks from right, toward head: Cham.

Thighs, cold and clammy: Calc. c. Merc. v.
——, fatigue in: Lyc.
——, heaviness and numbness of: Aloe.
——, tearing pains down: Rhus.

Toes, cramps of: Sec.
——, spread apart or bent backward: *Sec.*

Walk, slow in learning to: Bar. c. *Calc. c. Calc. ph. Caust.*

20. SLEEP.

Dreams of robbers in the house: *Natr. mur.*
——, tiresome: Asclep. Bapt. Cyclam. *Rhus.*

Sleep, caressed and fondled, only when: *Kreos.*
——, comatose: *Op.* Rhus, *Zinc.*
——, ——, with crying out: *Apis,* Hell.
——, crying out, during: *Apis, Bell.* Calc. c. Psor. Rheum, Stram. Zinc.
——, disturbed: Acet. ac. Apis, Arg. n. Asclep.

Bapt. *Bell*. Bor. Calc. ph. Cham. *Cina*, Cyclam. Kreos. *Merc. v.* Natr. mur. Petrol. Picric ac. Plant. Podo. Psor. Rheum, Rhus, Sabad. Sil. Stann. Zinc.

Sleep, erections priapismic, with: Picric ac.
——, eyes half closed, with: *Bell*. Bry. Ipec. Kreos. Lyc. *Podo*. Samb. Sulph.
——, fright on awakening, with: Ign. *Lyc*. Psor. Stram. Zinc.
——, grinding of teeth, with: *Cina*. Plant. Podo.
——, irritability on awaking, with: *Lyc*.
——, jerking and twitching of limbs and muscles, with: Ant. t. *Bell*. Bor. Cham. Ipec. *Rheum*, Zinc.
——, jerking through the whole body, with: Zinc.
——, moaning, with: *Bell*. Cham. Kreos. Podo. Stann.
——, mouth half open, with: Samb.
——, night terrors: *Kali brom*.
——, rocked, only while: *Cina*.
——, snoring: *Op*. Stram.
——, starting, with: Æth. *Bell*. Bor. Carbol. ac. Zinc.
——, sweat, with: *China*, Mur. ac. Nitr. ac. *Psor*.
——, ——, ——, on forehead, cold: *Merc. v*. *Sil*.
——, ——, ——, —— ——, hot: *Cham*.
——, with waking often: Asclep. Calc. c.

Cicuta, Cina, Lyc. Petrol. Sep. *Sulph.*

Sleep, with waking often, feeling too hot: Phos,

——, —— ——, at 3 **A. M.**: *Calc. c.* China, *Nux v.* Sep.

Sleepiness: Ant. c. Ant. t. Arg. n. Arn. Asclep. *Bell.* China, Corn. c. Gels. Hip. m. Ipec. *Nux mos. Op.* Petrol. Samb.

——, **daytime**: Agar. Calc. ph. Kali c. Merc. v. Mur. ac. Nux v. *Phos.* Podo. Psor. Rhod. Sabad. Samb. Sep. *Sulph.*

——, **eating, after**: Agar. *Nux. v. Phos.*

——, **with inability to sleep**: *Bell.* Chel. Natr. mur. *Op.* Samb. Sil.

Sleeplessness: Acon. Bapt. Caps. Cina, *Coff.* Coloc. Hyos. Iod. Op. Paul. Phos. Samb.

——, **at night**: Acet. ac. *Jalap. Kreos.* Merc. v. Mur. ac. Samb.

——, **day and night**: Psor.

——, **from hunger in evening**: Ign.

——, **with frightful visions**: Op.

Somnolency: Ant. t. Bell. Nux mos. Op. Phos. ac.

Sopor: *Apis, Bell.* Bor. Carbo v. Cicuta, *Nux mos. Op.* Sulph.

21. Fever.

a Chill.

Chill: Camph. Dig.

—— **mingled with heat**: Dig.

Chilliness: Arg. n. Asar. E. Bol. Camph. Cicuta, Corn. c. Dig. Elat. Kali brom. Merc. c.

Picric ac. *Puls.* Sabad. Sarsap. Sil. Sulph

Chilliness even when exercising: Sil.

——— when leaving the fire: Aloe.

Coldness: Æth. *Camph. Jatr. Laur. Tabac.*

Shuddering: Acon. Camph. Raph.

———, internal: Acon.

———, without coldness: Lach.

b. Heat.

Heat: *Acon.* Bapt. Carbol. ac. Colost. Corn. c. *Dulc. Gels.* Kali bich. Magn. c. *Stram.*

———, dry: *Acon.* Apis, Ars. *Bell. Dulc. Sulph.*

———, ———, when sleeping, with sweat on waking: Samb.

———, external, with chill: Dig.

———, internal, with external coldness: *Ars. Canth.*

———, with aversion to uncover: Nux v.

———, ——— violent throbbing of the Carotids: Bell.

Hot flashes: Bol. Ign.

c. Sweat.

Sweat: Acon. Benz. ac. Bol. *China,* Cicuta, Corn. c. Ferr. Ign.

———, absence of: *Alum. Graph.*

———, chilliness, with: Cicuta, Dig.

———, cold: Æth. Ant. t. Calc. c. *Camph.* Cupr. Hell. Jatr. Picric ac. *Sec.* Sulph. *Tabac.* Tereb.

———, covered parts, on: Acon.

———, exertion, during: China, *Merc. c. Psor.*

——, greenish: Ars.
——, night, at: *China*, *Merc v.* Phos. Phos. ac. *Psor.* Staph.
——, offensive: Arn. *Bapt.* Graph. *Merc. v. Sil.* Staph.
——, oily: *Merc. v.*
——, profuse: Jabor. Op. *Psor.* Stram.
——, ——, followed by several watery stools: Bell.
——, sleeping, when: *China*, Mur. ac. Nitr. ac. Phos. *Psor.*
——, ——, ——, with desire to uncover: Mur. ac.
——, sour-melling: *Merc. v. Sil.*
——, ——, with coldness of surface: Ferr.
——, sticky: Cham. *Merc. v.*
——, vomiting, with: Acon.
——, waking, when, with dry heat during sleep: Samb.
——, warm, on forehead: *Cham.* Merc. v.

d. PULSE.

Pulse, coming in long waves: Zinc.
——, failing: Ferr.
——, full: *Acon.* Bapt. *Gels. Op.*
——, hard: *Acon.* Æth. *Bell.* China.
——, imperceptible: *Ars.* Carbo v. Crotal. Kali brom. Laur. Tereb.
——, intermitting: Carbo v. Hell. Nitr. ac. Thuja.
——, —— every third beat: *Mur. ac.*

Pulse, irregular: China, Laur. *Tabac.* Thuja.
—, rapid: *Acon. Æth.* Ant. t. *Ars. Bell.* China, Jabor. Kali brom. Kreos.
—, slow: Cupr. *Dig.* Laur. Mur. ac. *Op.*
—, small: *Æth. Bell.* Cupr.
—, soft: Bapt. Cupr. Gels.
—, weak: Ant. t. Cupr. Cyclam. Dig. Kali brom. *Kali c.* Kreos. Merc. c. Mur. ac. *Tabac.*

22. Skin.

Skin, blue: *Cupr.* Sec. Verat.
—, cold: *Ars.* Calc. c. *Camph.* Canth. *Cupr.* Hell. Laur. Merc. c. Podo. Sec. *Verat.*
—, — and blue: Crotal.
—, —, at night: *Camph.*
—, —, without change of color: *Camph.*
—, cool: Nux mos.
—, dirty, greasy-looking, with yellow blotches: Psor.
—, dry: Acon. *Alum.* Apis, Ars. Bol. Calc. c. Graph. Nux mos. Sulph.
—, eruption, partially developed on: Psor.
—, folds, remaining when pinched: *Verat.*
—, harsh: Alum. Sulph.
—, hot: Acon. Apis, Ars. Bol. Calc. c.
—, itching of, as though fecal matter would pass through: Graph.
—, livid: Bor. Laur.
—, pale: Acet. ac. Bor.
—, red spots on, burning and itching: Agar.

Skin, red and blue spots on: Ars.
——, sallow: Bol. *Chel.* Con. Corn. c. *Dig.* Fluor. ac. *Merc. v.* Nux v. Podo. Sep.
——, shriveled: *Sarsap. Sec.*
——, waxen: Acet. ac.
——, wrinkled: *Sulph.* Verat.

23. GENERAL SYMPTOMS.

Alternation of chest and bowel symptoms: Dig.
Anasarca: *Apis, Ars.* China.
Ascites: *Apis, Ars.* Colch.
Attack, sudden, without apparent cause: Hyosc.
Automatic motion of one side of body: *Hell.*
Aversion to being covered (to heat): Camph. Sec.
Brain-f g: Picric ac. (Sabad.)
Bruised feeling of whole body: Amm. m. *Arn. Bapt.* Gamb. Hep. Merc. c. Staph.
Chlorosis: *Alum.* Cyclam. *Ferr. Graph. Lyc.* Nux v. *Puls.*
Collapse: *Ars.* Camph. Canth. *Carbo v.* Crotal. *Laur. Sec. Tabac.*
Cramps: Camph. Carbo v. Coccul. Crotal. **Cupr.** Iris v. *Jatr.* Phos. ac. *Podo. Sec. Sulph.* Verat.
Cyanosis: Dig.
Debility (languor): Acet. ac. Alum. Ang. Ant. t. Apis, Arg. n. Arn. Ars. Asclep. Benz. ac. Bor. Brom. Bry. Calc. c. Caust. *China,*

Coccul. Colch. Colost. Con. *Corn. c.* Dig.
Dulc. *Ferr.* Fluor. ac. Gamb. Graph. Iod.
Iris v. Kali bich. Kali brom. Kali c. Kali
nit. Lach. Lept. *Lyc.* Magn. c. Merc. v.
Mez. Mur. ac. Nitr. ac. *Nux mos.* Nux v.
Phos. Podo. *Psor.* Raph. Rum. Sabad. Sang.
Sec. Sep. Staph. Sulph. Sul. ac. Thuja,
Verat.

Dentition very painful: *Kreos.*

Desire to go into the open air: Lyc.

Ebullitions of blood: Amm. m.

Ecchymoses: *Arn.* Sarsap. *Sul. ac.*

Emaciation: Acet. ac. *Arg. n. Ars.* Bor. *Calc. c.*
Calc. ph. China, *Ferr.* Gamb. **Iod.** Kreos.
Lyc. Natr. mur. Nitr. ac. Nux v. Op.
Petrol. Phos. **Sarsap.** Sep. *Sil.* Sulph.
Thuja.

—— **of the neck: Natr. mur.** Sarsap.

Exhaustion (prostration): Ant. t. Apis, Arn.
Ars. Bapt. Benz. ac. Bis. Bol. *Camph. Carbo
v.* China, Coff. Colch. Con. Corn. c. Cupr.
Cyclam. Dulc. Elat. Ferr. Iris v. Kreos.
Lach. Merc. c. Merc. v. Mez. Mur. ac. Nuph.
Picric ac. Plant. *Sec. Sep.* Sulph. Sul. ac.
Tabac. Tarax. Tereb. *Thuja, Verat.*

——, **absence of:** Phos. ac.

——, **with warm surface:** Bis.

Expansion, feeling of, in various parts: Arg. n.

Fainting: *Ars.* Coccul. Laur. *Nux mos.* Op.
Tabac. Verat. Zinc.

GENERAL SYMPTOMS.

Fainting, on rising up: Acon. Bry. Op. Thromb.
Faintness: Camph. Lept. Merc. c. Raph.
Feels particularly well the day before an attack: Psor.
Glands swollen: Asaf. *Bar. c. Calc. ph. Cist.* Graph. Hep. *Merc. v.* Mur. ac. Natr. mur. Nitr. ac. *Staph. Sulph.*
Hydrocephaloid, threatened: Æth. Apis, Calc. c. *Calc. ph. China*, Ipec. Kali brom. Phos. *Sulph. Zinc.*
Jactitations: Kali brom.
Jar, every little, is painful: Bell.
Jaundice: Bol. *Chel.* Con. Corn. c. *Dig.* Kali c. Merc. v. Nux v. Podo.
Jerks: Valer.
——, convulsive, of single limbs: Ign.
Joints aching in: Bol.
Lethargy: *Bell. Nux mos. Op.*
Mucous membranes, dryness of: Alum.
Pains appear and disappear suddenly: Bell.
——, over-sensitiveness to: *Hep.*
Paralysis: Tabac.
Paralytic weakness: Amm. m.
Peristalsis, generally reversed: Asaf.
Petechiæ: *Arn.*
Restlessness: *Acon.* Arg. n. *Ars.* Bapt. Bell. Bol. *Canth. Carbo v. Cupr.* Dulc. *Iod. Kali brom.* Paul. Rheum, *Rhus.*
—— all night: *Jalap. Kreos.*
—— from 4 to 6 P. M.: *Carbo v.*
Rheumatism: Bar. c. Calc. ph. Rheum, *Rhod.*

Sensation, disagreeable through whole body, and nauseous taste: Crotal.
—— of trembling, without visible trembling: *Sul. ac.*
Shaking of body, as if from palsy: Kali brom.
Slide down in bed, tendency to: Mur. ac.
Smell of body, filthy, even after washing: Psor. Sulph.
—— —— stool follows him, as if he had soiled himself: Sulph.
Softness of the flesh: Podo.
Sour smell of body: Colost. *Hep. Magn. c. Rheum, Sul. ac.*
Spasms (convulsions): *Æth. Bell.* Canth Carbo v. *Cham.* Cicuta, *Cina, Cupr.* Hyos. Ign. Ipec. Kali brom. Laur. Op. Tabac. Zinc.
—— during dentition: *Calc. c.* Ign. *Zinc.*
——, with screaming, foaming at mouth, unconsciousness, throwing the arms about: Lyc.
Stammering: Merc. v.
Starts: Kali brom.
Stretching: Graph. Podo.
Stupor: Apis, Arg. n. Arn. Ars. Bapt. *Bell.* Camph. Hyos. *Nux mos. Op.* Sulph.
——, with twitching of muscles: *Sulph.*
Subsultus: Hyos.
Sudden shrieks: *Apis, Hell.*
Talk, slow in learning to: *Natr. mur.*
Termination of, coryza, catarrh, pains in

chest by diarrhœa: Sang.
Trembling: *Arg. n.* Merc. c. Valer. *Zinc.*
Trismus and tetanus: Camph.
Twitching of muscles: Ant. t. *Bell.* Bor. Cham. Ipec. *Rheum,* Sabad. Sulph. Valer. Zinc.
Yawning: Ant. t. Elat. Plant. Podo. *Staph.*

LIST OF AUTHORS

CONSULTED IN THE PREPARATION OF THIS WORK.

HAHNEMANN. Chronic Diseases.
JAHR. New Manual. Repertory.
LIPPE. Materia Medica.
HALE. Materia Medica.
MURE. Materia Medica.
METCALF. Homœopathic Provings.
GROSS. Comparative Materia Medica
POSSART. Arzneimittellehre.
BŒNNINGHAUSEN. Repertorium. Keuchhusten. Pocket Book.
RAUE. Pathology and Therapeutics.
GUERNSEY. Obstetrics and Diseases of Females and Children.
HARTMANN. Specielle Therapie Acuter und Chronischer Krankheiten. Spec. Therap. Kinderkrankheiten.
TESTE. Diseases of Children.
WILLIAMSON. Diseases of Women and Children.
CROSERIO. Obstetrics.
WELLS. Diarrhœa.
WOLF. Hom. Erfahrungen, Erstes bis fünftes Heft.
JOURNALS. Am. Hom. Review, Vol. I. to VI. Hahn. Monthly, Vol. I. to III. British Jour. of Hom., Vol. XXV. U. S. Med. and Surg. Jour., Vol. I. to IV. Monthly Hom. Review, Vol. VIII. Am. Jour. of Hom. Mat. Med., Vol. I. to II. New England Med. Gazette, Vol. I. to IV. Am. Hom. Observer, Vol. I. to VI. Medical Investigator, Vol. II. to VI. Ohio Med. and Surg. Reporter, a few numbers.

Western Hom. Observer, a few numbers. North Am. Jour. of Hom., Vol. V. and XIV. Proceedings of Am. Inst. of Hom., of N. Y. Hom. Med. Soc., of Mass. Hom. Med. Soc., a few volumes.

ADDITIONAL WORKS

CONSULTED IN THE PREPARATION OF THE SECOND EDITION.

ALLEN. Encyclopædia of Pure Materia Medica.
HERING. Condensed Materia Medica.
HERING. Guiding Symptoms.
HUGHES. Pharmacodynamics.
DUNHAM. Lectures on Materia Medica.
DUNHAM. Homœopathy the Science of Therapeutics.
BÆHR. Science of Therapeutics.
RAUE. Annual Records
LILIENTHAL. Homœopathic Therapeutics.
HOYNE. Clinical Therapeutics.
FARRINGTON. Supplement to Gross' Compara ive Mat. Med.
BURT. Characteristic Materia Medica.
LIPPE. Repertory.
JOURNALS. Hahn. Monthly, Vol. I. to XV. North Am. Jour. of Hom., Vol. XX. to XXVIII. Med. Investigator, Vol. IX. to XI. U. S. Med. Investigator, Vol. I. to X. N. Y. Jour. of Hom., Vol. I. to II., Amer. Jour. of Hom. Mat. Med., Vol. VI. to IX. Amer. Observer, Vol. IX. The Clinique, Vol. I. to II. Medical Counselor, Vol. I. to IV. Hahn. Hospital Reports. Trans. N. Y. Hom. Med. Soc. Trans. Penna. Hom. Med. Soc. Proceedings of Am. Inst. of Hom.

ADDITIONAL WORKS CONSULTED IN THE PREPARATION OF THE FOURTH EDITION.

ALLEN. General Symptom Register.
KNERR. Repertory of Hering's Guiding Symptoms.

INDEX.

Preface to First Edition	3
Preface to Second Edition	5
Editor's Preface	7
Preface to Third Edition	10
Preface to Fourth Edition	12
Character and Object of the Work	15
Selection of the Remedy	16
Administration of the Remedy	21

PART FIRST.

Remedies and Their Indications	23
1 Acetic acid	23
2 Aconite	24
3 Æsculus hippocastanum	25
4 Æthusa cynap.	26
5 Agaricus	28
6 Aloe	29
7 Alumina	32
8 Ammon. mur.	34
9 Angustura	35
10 Antimon. crud.	36
11 Antimon. tart.	37
12 Apis mel.	38
13 Argent. nit.	41
14 Arnica mont.	43
15 Arsenicum	45
16 Asafœtida	47
17 Asarum Europ.	49
18 Asclepias tuberosa	50
19 Baptisia tinct.	51
20 Baryta carb	52

INDEX.

21	Belladonna	53
22	Benzoic acid	55
23	Bismuthum	56
24	Boletus laricis	57
25	Borax	58
26	Bovista	59
27	Bromine	60
28	Bryonia	61
29	Calcarea carb.	67
30	Calcarea phos.	65
31	Camphor	67
32	Cantharis	69
33	Capsicum	70
34	Carbo veg.	71
35	Carbolic acid	73
36	Causticum	74
37	Chamomilla	75
38	Chelidonium maj.	77
39	China	78
40	Cicuta virosa	80
41	Cina	82
42	Cistus Can	82
43	Cocculus	83
44	Coffea	84
45	Colchicum	85
46	Colocynthis	87
47	Colostrum	89
48	Conium	89
49	Copaiva	90
50	Cornus circin.	91
51	Crotalus horridus	92
52	Croton tig.	93
53	Cubeba	95
54	Cuprum met.	96
55	Cyclamen	97
56	Digitalis	98
57	Dioscorea v.	99

INDEX.

58 Dulcamara 101
59 Elaterium 102
60 Ferrum met. 103
61 Fluoric acid 104
62 Gambogia 105
63 Gelsemium 107
64 Graphites 108
65 Gratiola off. 110
66 Helleborus niger. 111
67 Hepar sulph. 112
68 Hippomane man. 113
69 Hydrophobin 114
70 Hyoscyamus 115
71 Ignatia 116
72 Iodine 118
73 Ipecacuanha 119
74 Iris versicolor 121
75 Jaborandi 122
76 Jalapa 123
77 Jatropha curc. 123
78 Kali bich. 124
79 Kali brom. 126
80 Kali carb. 127
81 Kali nit. 128
82 Kreosotum 129
83 Lachesis 130
84 Laurocerasus 131
85 Leptandra 133
86 Lilium tig. 134
87 Lithium carb. 135
88 Lycopodium 135
89 Magnesia carb. 138
90 Mercurius corr. 139
91 Mercurius sol. (Merc. viv.) 141
92 Mezereum 143
93 Muriatic acid 144
94 Natrum carb. 146

INDEX.

95 Natrum mur. 147
96 Natrum sulph. 148
97 Niccolum 150
98 Nitric acid 151
99 Nuphar lut. 153
100 Nux moschata 153
101 Nux vomica 155
102 Oleander 157
103 Opium 157
104 Oxalic acid 158
105 Paullinia sorb. (Guarana) 159
106 Petroleum 160
107 Phosphorus 161
108 Phosphoric acid 164
109 Picric acid 165
110 Plantago 166
111 Plumbum met. 167
112 Podophyllum 168
113 Psorinum 170
114 Pulsatilla nig. 172
115 Raphanus sat. 173
116 Rheum 174
117 Rhododendron 175
118 Rhus tox. 176
119 Rumex crisp. 178
120 Sabadilla 179
121 Sambucus nig. 180
122 Sanguinaria Can. 181
123 Sarsaparilla 181
124 Scilla 182
125 Secale corn. 183
126 Sepia 185
127 Silicea 186
128 Stannum met. 188
129 Staphisagria 188
130 Stramonium 190
131 Sulphur 191

INDEX.

132 Sulphuric acid 194
133 Tabacum 195
134 Taraxacum 196
135 Terebinthina 196
136 Thrombidium 197
137 Thuja occ. 198
138 Valeriana 199
139 Veratrum album. 200
140 Zincum met. 202
141 Zingibe 203

PART SECOND.

REPERTORY—

    Pathological Names 205
    Character of the Stools 207
    Conditions of the Stools and of the Accompanying
        Symptoms 224
           a. Aggravations 224
           b Ameliorations 237
    Accompaniments of the Evacuations 239
        a. Before Stool 239
        b. During Stool 243
        c. After Stool 250
General Accompaniments 256
1 Mind and Mood 256
2 Head 260
3 Eyes and Ears 262
4 Nose 263
5 Face 263
6 Mouth 266
7 Throat 271
8 Œsophagus 272
9 Appetite 272
10 Eructations 278
11 Nausea and Vomiting 278
12 Stomach 282
13 Abdomen 284
14 Anus 288

15 Urine	289
16 Sexual Organs	292
17 Chest	292
18 Back and Neck	294
19 Extremities	295
20 Sleep	297
21 Fever	299
a. Chill	299
b. Heat	300
c. Sweat	300
d. Pulse	301
22 Skin	302
23 General Symptoms	303